Patricia Kelley, PhD

Developing Healthy Stepfamilies: Twenty Families Tell Their Stories

Pre-publication
REVIEWS,
COMMENTARIES,
EVALUATIONS...

"**P**atricia Kelley's book is a useful tool for both treating therapists and concerned step-parents. The blended family faces many unique challenges.

The book helps normalize the predictable stepfamily crises by giving real life examples of how well-functioning stepfamilies have coped with such nitty-gritty issues as discipline, family rules, and money.

The chapters on discipline and money management are especially useful. My blended family clients feel more hopeful about surviving step-parenthood after reading this book."

Judith Wagner, MAMFCT
Family Therapist and Trainer,
Private Practice Marriage,
Family, and Child Therapy,
Burlington, Iowa

More pre-publication
REVIEWS, COMMENTARIES, EVALUATIONS . . .

"**S**tepfamilies will find Dr. Kelley's book a valuable source of information and guidance on issues arising in their families. Many also will find inspiration and hope in the message that stepfamilies can be and often are high-functioning, as seen in this report on twenty such families. . . . Some very practical suggestions are offered about discipline, money management, division of responsibilities between birth-parent and step-parent, and relations with ex-spouses and their kinfolk.

Dr. Kelley presents not only her own research but thoughtfully relates her findings to other research literature on stepfamilies. She is careful not to over-generalize or jump to conclusions. The degree of scholarly expertise demonstrated by Dr. Kelley enhances the trustworthiness of her findings and interpretations. Social workers, psychologists, and other human service professionals will find Dr. Kelley's book a valuable resource in understanding the problems and strengths of stepfamilies. The book is refreshingly strength-focused."

Elam Nunnally, PhD
Associate Professor,
School of Social Welfare,
University of Wisconsin

"**D**r. Kelley's *Developing Healthy Stepfamilies* provides a rare opportunity to gain intimate knowledge about stepfamily issues. Research data is presented and made available to complement the writer's findings in the areas of discipline, family roles, money management, and family rituals and traditions. Readers come to realize, through the uniqueness of each stepfamily, the variety of successful approaches to universal family issues.

I was most interested in the families' varied accounts of handling discipline and money issues. A spectrum of possibilities was presented by these families which enables the reader to extrapolate some fresh ideas for working with client families, and indeed, their own families.

This book will appeal to stepfamily members and counselors alike, as it provides a wonderful inside look at the wide array of family issues and their management."

Susan Cohene, MSW, RSW
Principal Therapist,
Cohene & Associates,
Vancouver, British Columbia

The Haworth Press, Inc.

Developing Healthy Stepfamilies

Twenty Families Tell Their Stories

HAWORTH Marriage & the Family
Terry S. Trepper, PhD
Senior Editor

Developing Healthy Stepfamilies
Twenty Families Tell Their Stories

Patricia Kelley, PhD

The Haworth Press
New York • London • Norwood (Australia)

The Haworth Press, Inc., 10 Alice Street, Binghamton, NY 13904-1580

Library of Congress Cataloging-in-Publication Data

Kelley, Patricia, 1935-
   Developing healthy stepfamilies : twenty families tell their stories / Patricia Kelley.
     p. cm.
   Includes bibliographical references and index.
   ISBN 1-56024-888-2 (alk. paper)
   1. Stepfamilies–Case studies. I. Title.
HQ759.92.K45   1994
306.874–dc20
                                         93-40908
                                          CIP

CONTENTS

ABOUT THE AUTHOR

Patricia Kelley, PhD, is Professor and Director of the School of Social Work, University of Iowa, Iowa City. She also maintains a private practice in marriage and family therapy and agency consultation. Dr. Kelley is a past president of the Iowa Association for Marriage and Family Therapy, has testified before the U.S. Senate Sub-Committee on Family, Children, Drugs, and Alcoholism, and was a visiting scholar at the School of Social Studies at the University of South Australia. A member of the American Association for Marriage and Family Therapy, the National Association of Social Workers, and the Council on Social Work Education, she has published numerous articles on family therapy issues and is editor of the book *Uses of Writing in Psychotherapy,* (The Haworth Press, Inc., 1990).

Foreword

There have always been stepfamilies. However, the antecedent of most of these families has changed during the past 30 years from death of a spouse to parental divorce. This is an important change that has brought with it heightened emotions and new family tasks, as many parents and stepparents are involved in raising the children they share.

During this century American families have been studied, analyzed, and restudied. Unfortunately, the momentum has been toward looking at their shortcomings rather than their strengths. One cartoon captures well the outcome of this work: A large auditorium devoted to a conference of "Children of Normal Parents" has exactly two individuals in the audience. In addition to the tendency to see pathology in most families, the view that first-marriage families represent the ideal "intact" family form, with other types of families falling along a continuum toward deviancy and deficiency, leaves remarried couples and their children and stepchildren in an uncomfortable spot in the cultural hierarchy.

What a breath of fresh air Patricia Kelley has brought into the arena by looking closely at 20 well-functioning stepfamilies! Building on what has been learned about families in general and stepfamilies in particular, Patricia compares what these stepfamilies report with the findings of clinicians and researchers. The earlier stepfamily studies have been important in providing a foundation for thinking about these families, and, just as the strengths of first-marriage families and the concomitants of successful functioning have been considered more recently, this study is an important step away from viewing stepfamilies as defective two-parent households. Instead, they are seen as different from first-marriage families, with their own characteristic situations to address.

Fortunately, the field of stepfamily study and reporting has been shifting toward a more balanced perception of remarriage with children from previous relationships. The inquiry appearing in this book takes a deeper look at what the adults and children in "healthy" stepfamilies say about how their own families operate. By introducing the family members individually and revealing how they deal with discipline, family roles, money, relationships, and family rituals, Kelley provides a rich picture of the creativity and flexibility these subjects have brought to their families.

Six families are in therapy and 14 are not, although a few of those have been in the past. While there are several differences between these two subgroups, it is refreshing and heartening to read the work of an author who is not automatically equating therapy with unhealthy functioning. Certainly there are families in therapy who are not functioning as they would like. However, families fall along a continuum in this regard, and, as Patricia says, "families that are functioning well are not free of stress or problems, for they are part of life" (p. 4).

This book illustrates well the process of integrating a stepfamily, the value of humor and patience, and the richness that can unfold. It is interesting and full of fun.

The suggestions for others made by a number of the families were succinctly stated by one family member when she said that her first suggestions were "flexibility, flexibility, and flexibility." These words keep echoing in my mind as a challenge not only to stepfamilies, but to the concepts of all of us as we think about modern American families. May you appreciate and enjoy this book as much as I have.

Emily B. Visher, PhD
Cofounder, Stepfamily Association of America
Lincoln, Nebraska

Preface

This is a book of stories about living in stepfamilies; the focus is more on what does work than on what does not. Twenty families tell their stories and discuss such issues as discipline, money, relationships with ex-spouses and their families, and the development of new traditions. This is not a guidebook on what to do, but rather a book showing the many ways in which stepfamilies function. As a group, stepfamilies are different from biologically based families in form and function. It is important for the families, and for those working with them, to recognize and accept these differences as normal.

The stepfamily is the fastest-growing family form in America today, and so it is important to know more about it. My interest in stepfamilies comes from several sources. I teach family theory and family therapy at the University of Iowa, and I maintain a private practice in marriage and family therapy, where I see different issues for stepfamilies than for other families. While I have seen some thorny problems in stepfamilies, as well as in other families, I know that stepfamilies can function well. Until very recently, however, most research and popular writing on stepfamilies has focused on problems and on those families in treatment.

This book is an outgrowth of a study I conducted in which stepfamilies who believed they were functioning well, and also those who were in treatment for problems, were interviewed. In an effort to isolate commonalities among stepfamilies who were functioning well, 20 stepfamilies were interviewed intensively in their homes, and the interviews were videotaped. In analyzing the videotapes, I was struck by the richness of the data, much of which would be lost in the research report. Over and above their answers to specific questions, all of the families had interesting stories to tell. It therefore made sense to write a book telling their stories, in addition to the research article, and all of the families agreed.

In a sense, the real authors of this book are the 83 individuals in these 20 families who told their stories on video, so that others could learn from their experiences. Over the summer of 1990, Patricia Kostel, then a graduate student research assistant, and I drove to unknown parts of eastern Iowa and western Illinois to interview these volunteers in their homes. Those interviews were interesting and fun, and that was the most enjoyable part of this project. My thanks to those families. I also acknowledge and thank the University of Iowa School of Social Work, for providing me student research assistants for the project and for a grant to pay small stipends to each family; the University of Iowa, for providing me with a Developmental Leave in 1991 to analyze the data while a Visiting Scholar at the University of South Australia in Adelaide; and to the School of Social Studies in South Australia, for providing me with consultation, assistance, and resources while I was there.

Specific thanks go to Patricia Kostel, MSW, Beth Larsen, MSW, and Lary Belman, MSW, for their efforts on behalf of this project while graduate student assistants at the University of Iowa, and to Professor Ken Rigby and graduate student Glenda Inverarity of the School of Social Studies at the University of South Australia for consultation and data entry. I would also like to acknowledge the helpful suggestions of Emily Visher, cofounder of the Stepfamily Association of America, and Terry Trepper of Purdue University, editor of the Marriage and the Family series for Haworth Press. My thanks to both of them for their careful readings of this manuscript. My final thanks and acknowledgments go to my husband, Verne Kelley, and to our children and my stepchildren who along with my parents have taught me about family life.

These families will be introduced one by one in the second chapter, using pseudonyms and changing identifying information. In the following chapters, how these families deal with the issues of discipline, money, and relationships with former spouses will be addressed. These are all issues which present the biggest challenges to stepfamilies, and these are areas in which it is especially important to recognize and accept differences from biologically based families. In other chapters, the use of rituals and traditions to help these new families bond will be addressed, and family roles will be considered. In the latter discussion, who does what in the family to keep things running smoothly will be noted, and the differences from biologically based families will be underscored. In each chapter, ideas from the families will be summarized and specific stories will be used to illustrate certain points.

Last will be a chapter called "Suggestions for Others," which will consist of the families' responses to the question, "What suggestions do you have for others who are beginning a new stepfamily?" This question was a favorite of the families, and the one to which the greatest number of family members spoke. These families want to help others, and have definite ideas to pass on. Many talked into the camera as if the receiver of the suggestion would watch it directly, even though they knew that the tapes would be erased after analysis.

This book is written with the intention of disseminating information and increasing understanding about stepfamilies through the stories of several such families. Stepfamilies are different from biologically based families in form and function, and these differences need to be recognized as appropriate, not abnormal. The information in these stories is useful for stepfamilies, for their friends and relatives, and for the professionals working with them, such as teachers, clergy, physicians, and counselors. This book is useful, also, for students of family studies and family therapy, since the families' stories are connected to family theory concepts; the use of genograms for family discussion should be helpful. Further, it is hoped that this de-emphasis on problems will decrease the image of stepfamilies as problematic. Last, it is hoped that this book will be enjoyed as stories of human drama, action, humor, and love.

Patricia Kelley, PhD

Chapter 1

Introduction

This is a book about stepfamilies who are functioning well. So much that has been written on the subject has been about problems in these families. There are books for families telling them how to avoid these problems, and books for family counselors and therapists with suggestions for counseling these families. While some researchers have noted the strengths in stepfamilies (Bohannan and Yahraes, 1979; Coleman, Ganong and Gingrich, 1985; Crohn, et al., 1982; Duberman, 1975; Knaub, Hanna, and Stinnett, 1984; Peterson and Zill, 1986; Sager et al., 1983), most of the academic research on stepfamilies has been problem-focused and based on a clinical population, that is, families in treatment for problems. The research not based on the clinical population has, on the whole, studied the functioning of stepfamilies on several variables, using what Ganong and Coleman (1986) call the "deficit model," comparing their functioning to biologically based families and viewing the differences as negative.

Those books and research articles are important; they are drawn upon and cited in this book and a suggested reading list is included at the end. The focus of this book, however, is different; it is about what does work well for some stepfamilies. This is a book of stories about living in stepfamilies, summaries of the stories told by the families themselves. Twenty families in a variety of different stepfamily situations describe how they live, what works, and what does not work for them. Common themes are noted, but there are no guidelines or answers, since each family is unique and has its own pattern. These stories demonstrate that there are many ways of doing things, that if one plan does not work, another might.

STEPFAMILIES TODAY

There are many kinds of stepfamilies. For this book I will use a definition borrowed from Emily and John Visher, founders of the Stepfamily Association of America, and authors of many books on the subject. They define a stepfamily as "a household in which there is an adult couple, at least one of whom has a child from a previous relationship" (Visher and Visher, 1988, p. 9). I agree with this definition, which is broad enough to include families who have primary custody of the children and those who do not, couples who are married and couples who are not, couples who are a man and a woman as well as same-sex couples, couples with one biological parent or two, and where the parent has been divorced, widowed, or not previously married. While these types of families have differences among them, they also share some common differences from the traditional biologically based family upon which society has developed its norms. I hope that this book will be useful for all types of stepfamilies, but for this project I interviewed only married couples with at least one stepchild (not biologically related to one adult) living in the home at least 50 percent of the time. This limitation was important so that similar questions could be asked of all families and comparisons could be drawn from them. The issues for married couples who have primary custody are different in many respects. Even with this limitation, there are a variety of family types represented here.

In my practice I see different issues for stepfamilies than for other families. While I have seen problems in stepfamilies, as well as in other families, I also know that stepfamilies can function well. In a study conducted of adolescents who were treated in out-patient mental health services (Kelley, Kelley, and Williams, 1989), only about half of the adolescents lived in single-parent or stepfamily situations. On the basis of some of the literature on the subject (Nunn, Parish, and Worthing, 1983; Wallerstein, 1985), I expected a higher rate of children of divorce represented in the clinical population. Yet, other literature suggested little difference in adjustment between children in biologically based or stepfamilies (Duberman, 1975; Santrock et al., 1982). More current research has emphasized the many factors that affect good adjustment (Hetherington et al.,

1989). Thus, I became interested in those families who clinicians do not see and who are rarely written about: those stepfamilies who believe that they function well. Then I began to wonder, what are the elements of good functioning in stepfamilies? Several studies have isolated the variables of healthy family functioning (Beavers and Hampson, 1990; Epstein, Baldwin, and Bishop, 1983; Epstein, Bishop, and Levin, 1978; Olson, Sprenkle, and Russell, 1979), but the applicability of those variables to stepfamilies has not been tested. Other authors have stressed the importance of recognizing the differences in stepfamily structure and rules (McGoldrick and Carter, 1988; Visher and Visher, 1979, 1985, 1988; White and Booth, 1985; Sager et al., 1983; Schwebel, Fine, and Renner, 1991), but these differences were not empirically tested. The interviews discussed in this book are an outgrowth of an exploratory project to look at those differences.

The stepfamily is an important family form to study and understand, since it is believed to be the fastest-growing family form in the United States in the 1990s. The divorce rates in the United States grew rapidly in the 1970s and leveled off in the 1980s; 79 percent of the men and 75 percent of the women remarry, and about 60 percent of these adults have children (Glick and Lin, 1986). If you add to these numbers those families where one parent has died, or where a parent had not married at all, the large number of stepfamilies becomes apparent. Glick and Lin (1986) estimated that one in five children under 18 is a stepchild, and that this type of family will outnumber all others by the year 2000.

Although the stepfamily form is becoming normative, most of the people in these families were raised to view the proper family form as the biologically based family, and have tried to model their families after that traditional form. Most family theorists and researchers have recognized that stepfamilies have different forms and functions, and that their attempts to replicate the nuclear biologically based family can and has created problems (Johnson, 1980; Mills, 1984; Sager et al., 1983; Visher and Visher, 1979, 1985, 1988). The recognition and validation of a different family form by the stepfamilies and by their surrounding support institutions such as churches, schools, and work places is important.

Attempts have been made in recent years to normalize these

families by using different names to decrease the bad connotation. Thus, we have heard the words "Blended" (Poppen and White, 1984), "Re-married" (McGoldrick and Carter, 1988), "Bi-nuclear" (Ahrons and Rodgers, 1987) (this term does have a slightly different meaning, see Chapter 6 for further discussion), and even "Re-constituted" (Robinson, 1980). However, since such families consist of stepmothers, stepfathers, and stepchildren, the term "stepfamilies" makes the most sense, and is clearest. There seems to be a recent trend to use the term "step" again. I support this trend, and believe that we can aim now to change the image by making the term respectable instead of changing it.

HEALTHY FAMILY FUNCTIONING

The concept of healthy or good family functioning is relative, but it needs to be addressed and defined here since this project is based on an assumption that such distinctions can be made. Certainly families that are functioning well are not free of stress or problems, for they are part of life. The idea of seeing families as either healthy or dysfunctional is not one that I find useful. Most family theorists and researchers agree that family functioning is a continuum, not distinct categories, and that there are several variables to assess along that continuum (Beavers and Hampson, 1990; Epstein, Baldwin, and Bishop, 1983; Epstein, Bishop, and Levin, 1978; Olson, Sprenkle, and Russell, 1979). The findings of these researchers have proven useful as a way to view families, and such a view makes sense theoretically.

In my experience, family competence is a multifaceted continuum and families change over time as to where they fall on this continuum. These changes come about, planned or unplanned, through events, passage of time, and circumstance. In this view, families are not functional or dysfunctional, for that locks them into place, at least in the mind of the labeler. Families act in more- or less-functional ways at different times under different circumstances. How a family responds to a particular situation depends on the view that family has about the meaning of that event, on where the family is in its life cycle when the event occurs (McGoldrick and Carter, 1988), and on other stressors (any change) at the time of the event. In other words, one family may react more negatively than another to one event, but at a different time, or on a different issue at the same time, the other family might react more negatively.

For reasons of biology and environment, some families seem to withstand overall pressure better than others, while some families seem to function at a lower level more of the time. Families can and do change; if I did not believe this, I would not be a family therapist. All families have strengths and all families have problems. I believe that the emphasis on dysfunctional families has led some families and some therapists into an over-focus on problems and an under-focus on the strengths, which skews the view of reality and keeps the families stuck in the sick role. Furthermore, such labels presume one right way of being. There are a wide range of family patterns which vary by individual family and also by cultural background; it is not respectful to hold up one way of being as a model for all families.

As a basis for assessing these families in this project, I have used the model and the scales of Beavers and Hampson (1990). They view family functioning in terms of the qualities of the relationships, communication, and exchanges; they see all families as falling on a progressive continuum rather than into categorical types; and they assume a potential for growth and adaptation. They also recognize that families at similar competence levels may have different styles of interacting and relating, and that these styles may also change over time, as the system develops and the individuals mature. Furthermore, these theorists outline the variables of family functioning, recognizing that most families are higher or lower on different variables. The variables that they address are: Structure, how the family allocates power and enforces rules, how close the members are to each other, what coalitions exist, and how flexible the coalitions and roles are; mythology, how family members view themselves and how congruent these views are with views of outsiders; negotiation, how efficient they are in problem solving; autonomy, how much individuality is allowed and expressed without losing closeness or support of each other; clarity of expression; and affect, how broad a range of emotions are allowed and expressed, the degree of expressed empathy, and the overall mood and tone of the family.

THE FAMILIES

Who are these families and how did they come to be interviewed for this project? This book is an outgrowth of a study of healthy stepfamily functioning, in which stepfamilies who defined themselves as functioning well were interviewed, and common threads were assessed (Kelley, 1992). Stepfamilies who were receiving services from family counseling agencies were also interviewed using the same schedule of questions, and differences between the two groups were noted. In addition to the interviews, which were videotaped, a standardized test of family functioning was administered to determine if the difference between the two groups was real, and it was. These differences are discussed in Chapter 2. In analyzing the videotapes, I was struck by the richness of the data, much of which would be lost in the research report. Over and above their answers to specific questions, all of the families had interesting stories which they were anxious to share with others.

Families were recruited for this project from throughout eastern Iowa and western Illinois in several ways. First, families who consider themselves as functioning well were recruited through a newspaper advertisement, discussion on a radio show, church bulletins, announcements at conferences on families, and persons conducting groups for stepfamilies. In all of these situations I noted that I was looking for stepfamilies who considered themselves to be functioning well for a study of healthy family functioning in stepfamilies. Then, to recruit the "service" families, those being served by agencies at the time, I placed fliers in the waiting rooms of six agencies serving families, so families could volunteer with no knowledge or coercion from the staff. When there were few such volunteers, agency staff did mention the study to clients. For recruitment into both the high-functioning and service groups, a small stipend was offered to each family in hopes of having a broad economic representation.

Although I aimed at diversity of the families for the study, certain parameters had to be set so there would be some basis for comparison. As noted earlier, only families where the adult couple in the home was married and where there was at least one child who was a stepchild to one of the adults, and who was living in the home at least half of the time, were recruited. This decision does not negate the importance of other forms of stepfamilies, but the issues are so different for unmarried couples and for families who do not have primary custody of children that findings would not be comparable. This decision, however, did reduce diversity. These families are heavily drawn from the middle and upper-middle socioeconomic classes, for both groups. Staff from agencies who serve predominantly lower-income clients told me that few of their families remarry, often for economic reasons.

The highest number of volunteers came from church bulletins; that method reached a large number of people, and they seemed willing to help. In some situations, the minister or rabbi suggested to a family that they volunteer. Their referral as a high-functioning family was viewed as a compliment by many family members. It is interesting to note that though the media generated several inquiries, none of the families in the study were recruited by this method. In all, 20 families were interviewed; 14 who were recruited as high functioning and six from the population receiving clinical services. After family members contacted me as potential volunteers, I interviewed them by phone to ensure that they met the criteria and to explain the procedures to them. I did lose several families through this process; a few were not appropriate for this study because the stepchild was no longer living at home, the couple had not yet married, or, in two situations, the adults who contacted me had been raised in stepfamilies but were not living in one now. I acknowledged that they knew the subject well, but I was looking for families with an immediate perspective. Others chose not to participate when they found out that the interviews would be videotaped, and in several situations one family member agreed to participate and the idea was vetoed by a spouse or child. I asked that all persons living in the home 50 percent or more of the time be present for at least part of the interview. All of the families complied with this request, although small children were not required to stay for the entire interview. Some parents gave the incentive money to the adolescents to gain compliance. Most of the families that were interviewed enjoyed the process and said so. Only one family, a service family, seemed overtly stressed by the process. The rate of drop out (those who agreed to participate and changed their minds before the interview) was about twice as high for the service families as for the high-functioning families, with a ratio of five to two.

The interviews were conducted in the families' homes, except for two situations where the families chose to come to my office. I conducted all of the interviews following an interview schedule, but allowed time for free discussion and recommendations from the family. A graduate student, as a research assistant, videotaped the interviews, asked questions of her own, and requested clarification on some points. The average length of the interviews was 1 1/2 hours, and they often assumed a social and festive air as the families enjoyed discussing themselves. Since the focus of the interviews was not on problems but on what worked and what did not, very few of the families in either group responded with caution or defensiveness. While there was serious discussion, the interviews were lively, with good humor prevailing.

The remainder of this book introduces you to the families and summarizes their interviews. I hope that you find their ideas on a variety of topics useful, and that you enjoy their stories.

Chapter 2

The Families

In this chapter, the families are introduced, first individually and then as a group. The 20 families are given names alphabetically, to aid the reader in remembering which family is which as their ideas are discussed in the following chapters. The names are chosen at random, to fit alphabetically and are not meant to represent any aspect of the family, nor are the names similar to their real names in any way. Generally, ideas distilled from these families' stories will be summarized around common themes and ideas; specific stories will also be used to highlight certain examples.

These families represent diverse family structures and a range of situations. They lack the ethnic diversity I had hoped for, but there is a wide range of income levels, from a family living in public housing to two families with incomes over 80,000 dollars, even though the families were clustered in the middle ranges. These are all midwestern families; most are drawn from three larger urban areas, with a few each from the small university community where I am based and from the surrounding rural area. For this book, the families from the university town are included in the urban category, to distinguish them from the rural communities.

Fourteen of these families were recruited as "high functioning" by self-definition, and six were recruited from counseling agencies serving families; they are referred to as high-functioning and service families in this book. The structure of each family will be referred to as simple (only one partner was previously married or had a child by a previous relationship) or complex (both partners were previously married or had children by a previous relationship). A "stepfather family" consists of a mother, her biological children, and a stepfather, and a "stepmother family" includes a stepmother, a father, and his biological children. For further discussion of these factors, please see the demographic section at the end of this chapter.

MEET THE FAMILIES

The first 14 families were referred to this project as high functioning.

The Allen Family

The first family lives in an urban area, having recently moved from another part of the country. They represent a simple stepfather family, where a never-married man married a divorced woman with two sons, and they now have a mutual daughter. The Allens did not sign a form releasing specific information and genogram material, but they understand that their stories will be told and incorporated into discussions throughout the book.

The Butterworth Family

The Butterworths represent a simple stepmother family and live in an urban area. Mrs. Butterworth is 24 years old and never previously married, whereas Mr. Butterworth was married for 11 years to his first wife. This family also has two boys from his previous marriage and a mutual daughter, 18 months old. The couple has been married a little over two years. They both have high school diplomas; the husband is a skilled laborer who earns a good salary, and the wife does not work outside of the home. This family functioned well in spite of a severe stressor in that one of the boys has a life-threatening illness and requires a great deal of care. The stepmother, the boy's biological mother, and the maternal grandparents all share in his care, which binds the potential adversaries together in an unusual way. The father has primary custody, but his ex-wife shares in child care and has the boys frequently. The couple was referred by their minister as "healthy."

The Butterworth Family

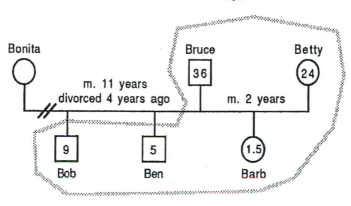

The Campbell Family

The Campbell family lives in a rural area, and represents a complex stepfamily. They have been married for eight years. Mr. Campbell was previously married and divorced twice, each marriage lasting for five years, with no children. Mrs. Campbell was also previously married for 13 years, and had three children. One daughter and a son currently live with the Campbells; the oldest daughter is married. The children's father lives out of state. Mr. Campbell works as a skilled laborer, and has a high school diploma. Mrs. Campbell has a bachelor's degree and is a full-time professional. The family learned of the study through their church bulletin.

The Campbell Family

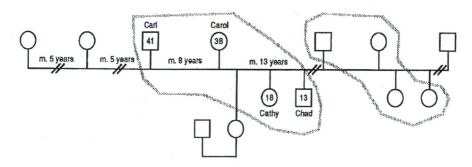

The Davis Family

The Davises are an urban family that represents the complex stepfamily. The couple has been married for two years. Each was previously married once and both have children from those marriages. Mrs. Davis was married for 15 years. Her son lived with his father after the divorce five years ago, and now attends college. Her daughter lives in the Davis household. Mr. Davis, married for 11 years, has a daughter and a son, who both live in another state with their mother. They visit the Davis home in the summertime. Mr. and Mrs. Davis have graduate degrees and work as salaried professionals. Mrs. Davis read about the study in their church bulletin, and volunteered to participate.

The Davis Family

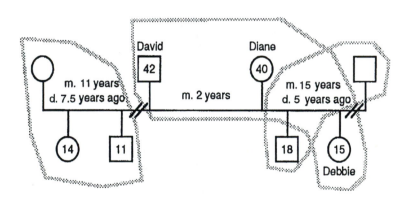

The Evans Family

The Evans family is a simple stepmother family, living in an urban area. They have been married for ten months. Mrs. Evans was not married previously. Mr. Evans was married twice before, both times for a period of five years. He has primary custody of his eight-year-old son from the second marriage. His second wife has remarried and lives out of state, and their son spends time with her in the summer. Both Mr. and Mrs. Evans are doctoral-level professionals. The family was referred to the study by their minister.

The Evans Family

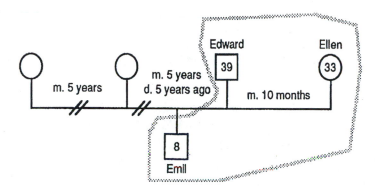

The Foster Family

The Fosters live in an urban area, and have been married for nine years. They represent a simple stepmother family. Mr. Foster has two children from a previous marriage of 6 1/2 years. This is Mrs. Foster's first marriage. Mr. Foster's children spend half-time in each parent's household, changing households every week. Both Mr. and Mrs. Foster have graduate degrees and work as full-time professionals. The Foster's minister recommended them for the study.

The Foster Family

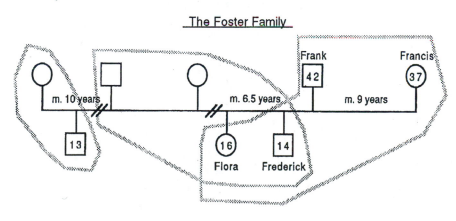

The Gardner Family

Mr. and Mrs. Gardner have been married four years and live in an urban area. Representing a complex stepfamily, they each have children from previous relationships, and a mutual daughter, age 2 1/2. Mrs. Gardner's six-year-old son lives in the Gardner household and has no contact with his biological father. Mr. Gardner, previously married for 11 years, has a young adult son living out of the home. They are both bachelor-level professionals. Mr. Gardner works outside of the home, and Mrs. Gardner has a day-care business in the home. The family was recommended by a friend who was participating in the study.

The Gardner Family

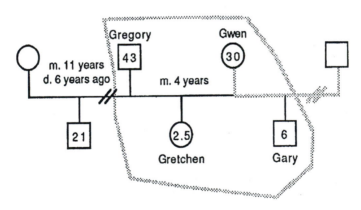

The Hall Family

The Halls reside in a rural area, and are an example of a simple stepfather family. They have been married for 14 years, and have an 11-year-old daughter. Mrs. Hall has primary custody of a son, age 17, from a previous marriage of three years. Her son has only occasional contact with his biological father. Mr. Hall has had some college, and owns a small business. Mrs. Hall has a bachelor's degree, and works as a salaried professional. The Halls learned about the study through a professional organization.

The Hall Family

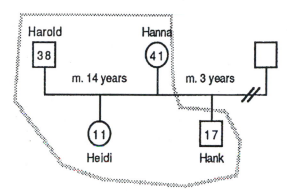

The Ibsen Family

The Ibsen family is a complex stepfamily, living in an urban area. They have been married one month. Mr. Ibsen was previously married for 19 1/2 years, and has two children from that marriage. His 20-year-old daughter is in college and is home part time; his 10-year-old son has lived with him since the divorce one year ago. Mrs. Ibsen was previously married for five years, but had no children. Both Mr. and Mrs. Ibsen have bachelor's degrees. Mrs. Ibsen works as a salaried professional, and Mr. Ibsen is employed in the field of business. The Ibsens heard about the study through a professional colleague.

The Ibsen Family

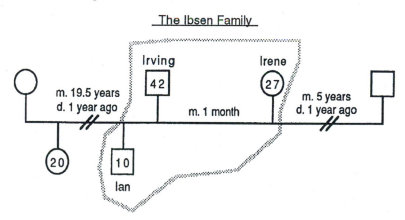

The Jones Family

The Jones family lives in an urban area, and represents a complex stepfamily. They have been married for 2 1/2 years, and both were previously married. Mr. Jones was married for 17 years, and has a daughter, age 11, from that marriage. Mrs. Jones was married for 18 years, but has no children. Mr. Jones's daughter lives half-time in each of her parent's households. Mr. and Mrs. Jones are both self-employed professionals with graduate degrees. The family learned of the study through a professional association.

The Jones Family

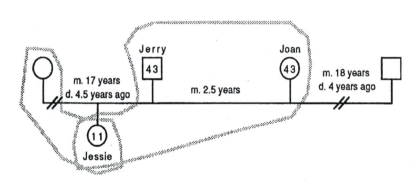

The Klein Family

The Klein family represents a simple stepfather family, and lives in a rural area. They have been married for 11 years, and have a 10-year-old son. This is Mr. Klein's first marriage. Mrs. Klein was previously married for 3 1/2 years. Her 13-year-old daughter from that marriage lives in the Klein household. Mr. Klein has a high school diploma, and works in a factory. Mrs. Klein has a high school diploma and received some technical training after high school. She is temporarily unemployed. The Kleins heard about the study from a friend who was participating.

The Klein Family

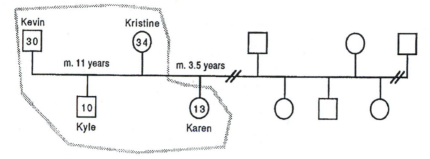

The Lange Family

The Langes represent a complex stepfamily, and live in an urban area. They have been married for nine years. Mr. Lange has been married twice before, the first time for five years, and the second for 13 years. He has four daughters from these marriages, as well as some grandchildren. The youngest daughter attends college, and is in and out of his home. Mrs. Lange was married once before, for 8 1/2 years. She has two sons from that marriage, ages 15 and 13. Both boys live in the Lange household, and have had no contact with their father since his remarriage a few years ago. Both Mr. and Mrs. Lange have had some college education, and are employed in business. The Langes heard about the study through friends.

The Lange Family

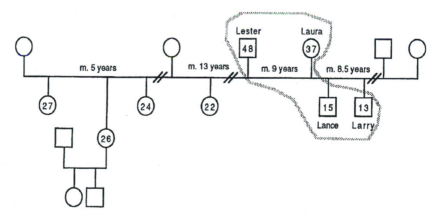

The Martin Family

The Martins, married for two years, represent a simple stepfather family. They reside in an urban area. This is Mr. Martin's first marriage, and Mrs. Martin's second. Mrs. Martin has a daughter, age 14, from her first marriage of four years. Her daughter lives in the Martin household, having no contact with her biological father. For the first year of their marriage, the Martins also had a friend's teenage son living with them. Mr. Martin is employed as a doctoral-level professional. Mrs. Martin had three years of college and works as a secretary. The family learned about the study from a speech.

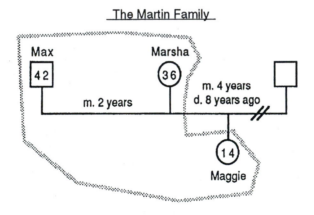

The Martin Family

The Nolan Family

The Nolans represent a complex stepfamily, and live in an urban area. They have been married for two years. They have a nine-month-old son, and each brings children from former marriages. Mr. Nolan was widowed after 20 years of marriage. They had three children, one girl and two boys, ages 17, 14, and ten. Mrs. Nolan had been married for four years when her husband left. She has a six-year-old daughter and a four-year-old son from that marriage, who have no contact with their biological father. Both Mr. and Mrs. Nolan are professionals with advanced degrees. The Nolans learned about the study through a professional association.

The Nolan Family

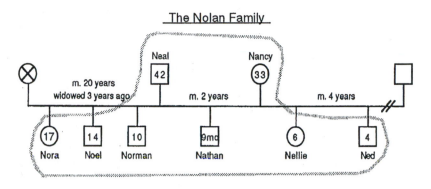

The following six families were recruited through social agencies serving families.

The Owen Family

The Owens represent a complex stepfamily, and live in an urban area. They have been married for seven years, both with previous marriages. Mr. Owen was married for 31 years, and has two daughters who live out of the home. The oldest daughter is married, and has a child. Mrs. Owen has a 17-year-old son from her former marriage of 3 1/2 years. Her former husband left when their son was an infant, and has had no contact with him since that time. Mr. Owen legally adopted Mrs. Owen's son, who resides in the Owen household. Mr. Owen has a high school diploma, and some technical training. He is currently employed as a skilled technician. Mrs. Owen has a bachelor's degree, and is employed part time in professional work.

The Owen Family

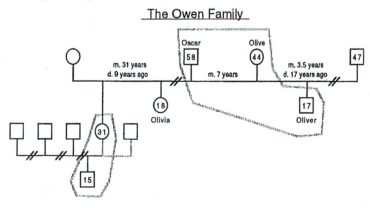

The Peterson Family

The Peterson family lives in an urban area, and represents a complex stepfamily. Mr. and Mrs. Peterson have been married for seven months, each has been married before, and both bring children to the home. The Petersons did not sign a form releasing specific information and genogram material, but they understand that their stories will be told and incorporated into discussions throughout the book.

The Rogers Family

The Rogers family is a complex stepfamily, living in an urban area. They have been married seven months, both having been married before. Mr. Rogers has three children and two grandchildren from his first marriage. His two daughters are adults and living out of the home, and his son, age 11, lives in the home. Mrs. Rogers had three previous marriages. Her 18-year-old son is in the process of moving out of the home, and her 15-year-old son lives in the home. Both Mr. and Mrs. Rogers have high school diplomas and work as skilled technicians. He is employed full time, and she works part time.

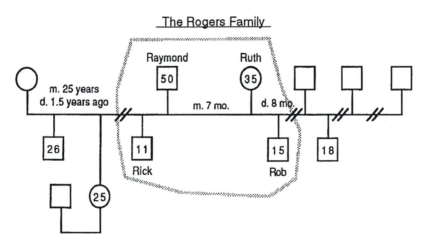

The Rogers Family

The Smith Family

The Smiths live in an urban setting, and represent a complex stepfamily. They have been married for one year, each bringing children to the family from previous marriages. Mrs. Smith has primary custody of a daughter, age 13, and a son, age 12. The children's father resides in another state, so they see him once a year. Mr. Smith has children from both of his previous marriages. His young adult son lives out of the home, while his son and daughter, ages 11 and nine, reside with their mother. Both Mr. and Mrs. Smith have bachelor's degrees, and are salaried professionals.

The Smith Family

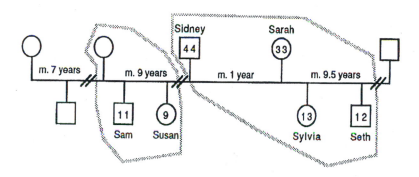

The Taylor Family

The Taylor family represents a complex stepfamily, and resides in a rural community. They have been married for 16 months. Each was previously married, and brings children to the family from those marriages. Mr. Taylor was married twice, for seven and two years. He has a daughter, age 18, and a son, age 16, from his first marriage, of whom he has primary custody. Mrs. Taylor was married for seven years, and has a son, age 9 1/2. He also resides in the Taylor household. Both Mr. and Mrs. Taylor have high school educations, and Mrs. Taylor has vocational training. Both are employed full time.

The Taylor Family

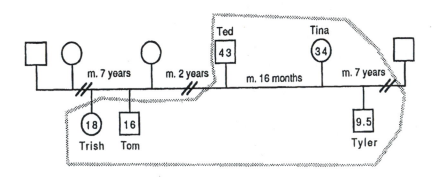

The Wilson Family

The Wilsons live in an urban area, and represent a complex stepfamily. They have been married for five years, each bringing children to the home from previous marriages. Mrs. Wilson was married for 13 years, and has primary custody of a 17-year-old son. Her son has little contact with his biological father, who lives far away. Mr. Wilson shares custody of his 12-year-old son, who lives half-time in each parent's household. Mr. Wilson's two adult daughters live outside of the home. Both Mr. and Mrs. Wilson have graduate degrees. Both are employed as full-time professionals.

The Wilson Family

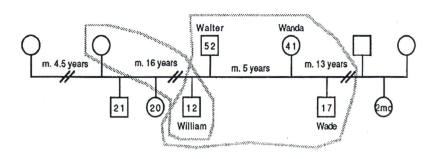

DEMOGRAPHIC INFORMATION
AND GROUP DESCRIPTION

Now that the families have been introduced, they will be presented as a group, and demographic factors will be noted. Generally they will be viewed as a group of 20. However, at times they will be looked at as two groups: high functioning and service. This distinction will be made when there is an important difference between them as groups.

First, it is important to determine if the difference between the high-functioning and service groups is real; that is, are the high-functioning families better functioning? The difference between these two groups was validated through use of a standardized instrument developed by Beavers and Hampson (1990), which contains a self-rating inventory completed by both the husband and wife, and an outsider rating scale based on four raters observing segments of the videotapes. The ratings of the husbands, wives, and raters correlated well with each other, and statistically significant differences were found between the two groups. For further information on statistical findings, please see Kelley (1992).

Although differences were found between the two groups, the 20 families fall along a continuum of family functioning from those with several problems to families functioning very well. Beavers and Hampson (1990) found that about 67 percent of families in the general population fall into the midrange category on their scale of health/competence, with 16 percent of the population falling above and 16 percent falling below that range. On this scale, these families ranged from below midrange to the top end of the adequate range (only 2 percent of the population would fall above the adequate range). None of the families fell into the severely dysfunctional range. The average of the service group fell at the low end of the midrange category, and the high-functioning group average was in the middle of the adequate range (highly functional). As a total group they represent families who function better than the average family in the general population. (See Figure 1.)

Except for a few categories, which are noted, the service and high-functioning groups did not differ on demographic factors. The fact that these two groups are similar demographically and are

Figure I: S.F.I Scores of Wives

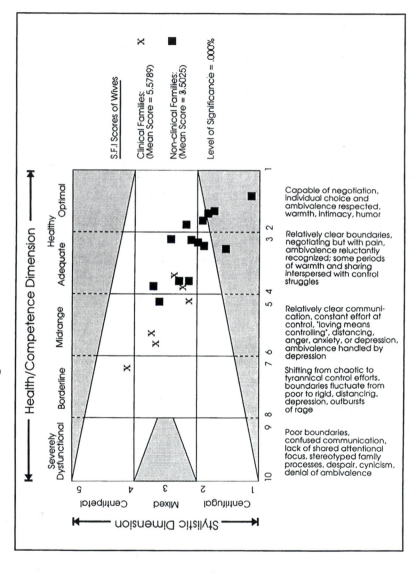

different in degree of family functioning, will make the comparisons on their ideas and practices useful. Yet, it is important to keep in mind that all of these families are relatively high functioning. As a study of healthy family functioning, the emphasis in all of the interviews was on what works. Recognizing this point, the comparisons of the highly functioning stepfamilies to those with more problems can be instructive.

The age of the wives in this group of 20 range from 24 to 44, with the average at 35.4. The range for the husbands was 30 to 58, with the average at 42.6. One difference between the groups was found here; the men in the service group were significantly older than men in the high-functioning group (47.5 to 40.3), and there was a bigger age difference between spouses in the service group (11 years to six in the high-functioning). There was not a significant difference in the wives' ages by group.

The education range for both husbands and wives was from less than high school to doctorate, with most having a bachelor's degree. There was not a difference between the groups on this factor, but in both groups the men were somewhat more educated than the women (slightly more than a college degree to slightly less). The group as a whole is more educated than the population in general. Likewise, the range of jobs and incomes was broad, but the group as a whole had higher-level jobs and incomes than the general population. The jobs ranged from unskilled labor to what I classified as Professional I, which included physicians, professors, and attorneys. The largest number fell into the classification Professional II, which included teachers, nurses, engineers, and social workers. The family incomes ranged from the category of under 15,000 dollars to over 80,000 dollars, with the average at about 45,000 dollars. While this figure is higher than the average family income, in most of these stepfamilies both partners are employed out of the home. Only two of the 20 families, one in each group, had a parent staying home full time to care for house and children.

Differences were not found between the groups on the number of previous marriages nor on the length of those marriages. For the group of 20, the number of previous marriages ranged from zero to three for the wives and zero to two for the husbands. The length of those marriages ranged from three to 13 years for the wives and two to 31 for the husbands.

Family structure is a variable which several researchers have found to be significant in adjustment of stepfamilies (Clingempeel and Brand, 1985; Clingempeel, Brand, and Ievoli, 1984; Ihinger-Tallman and Pasley, 1986). Usually, the more complex the family structure, the more difficulty there is in the stepfamily adjustment. There are many varieties of stepfamilies, but, as noted earlier, I chose to divide the families into two groups, simple and complex, since there are only 20 families represented here. A main difference between the types is the number of relationships and extended families that need to be managed. While the many potential relationships may be a benefit for the children in that they represent more sources of support and love, they can also mean the potential for more conflict.

All six of the service families here fall under the complex category, and, in four out of the six, children from both partners were living in the home (two had the wives' children only). In the high-functioning group, seven families were simple stepfamilies, four with stepfathers and three with stepmothers, and seven were of the complex variety, but in all but two of these complex families children from only one of the partners were living in the home. In three of these families only the mothers' children were in the home while the fathers' children were either grown and on their own, or living with the biological mother. Two of these families had wives who had been married before but had not had children; the children here were the husbands'. There is a difference between the two groups here, and it is obvious that when there are fewer relationships to manage the adjustment is easier. The total number of children in the home did not differ by group (the range was one to six with the average being two in both groups), but having children from both partners did seem to make a difference.

The other factor which seemed to make a difference was the length of the present marriage. The high-functioning group had been married longer, on the average (5.4 years), than the service group (2.8 years). This makes sense, of course; those families having more problems are less likely to stay together. However, it also seems to be true that this is a developmental matter, that there are problems in adjustment in the beginning of a stepfamily, which may decrease over time. Several of the high-functioning families noted that they had sought counseling for problems in earlier years as a stepfamily, and their main suggestion now was "patience." They all said that things had to be sorted out at first and that time had indeed been a main factor in their success.

Some studies have found that having a mutual child has a positive effect on stepfamilies (Bernstein, 1989), although again the circular effect could be operating in that the families who feel that they are functioning well are more likely to have children. The numbers of these families having a mutual child was small; six families had one mutual child and none had more than one. It is interesting to note that all six of the families with a mutual child were high-functioning. Of course, since the service families had not been married as long, perhaps some of them will have a child in the future.

The last demographic factor assessed here is whether there are children living out of the home. Twelve of these 20 families had no children out of the home. Of the eight families who had children living out of the home, the age range of the youngest was nine to 22, and the age range of the oldest was 14 to 31. Some of these "children" were in the custody of another parent, but most had left home, as adults, to attend school or to live on their own or in their own newly formed families.

In summary, these 20 families represent a wide range of stepfamily types, with some diversity of income and life style. As a group, they look like typical families except that their incomes and educations are higher than in the general population.

Chapter 3

Discipline

Discipline has been defined as "training that develops self-control, character, or orderliness and efficiency" (*Webster's*, 1980). Here, the term is used to describe the manner in which family rules are enforced, and the style of leadership exerted by parents. Discipline has been noted to be a major source of tension for stepfamilies (McGoldrick and Carter, 1988; Visher and Visher, 1988). Although this book is not meant to focus on problems, areas which may be problematic need to be addressed, and ways in which these challenges have been met by families who are functioning well can be instructive.

There are societal and familial expectations which increase the difficulties in the area of child discipline. When men with children remarry they often expect the new wife to be the mother to their children. This expectation is an unrealistic one which, as noted by Carter (1989), has led to the wicked stepmother image which has prevailed over time. In earlier times, a single father was more often widowed, and would remarry so the children would have a mother, as if she were a replaceable part. Being a mother means nurturing, disciplining, and loving. Children often resent a new woman as a replacement for their mother, and do not act lovable or accept discipline, so the woman is viewed as a bad mother for her failure. After a while, the stepmother may believe that she is a bad mother because she did not love these children instantly, and they did not accept her attempts to love or discipline them. Since being a good mother has been a main source of acceptance by self and others for many women, and being in charge of emotional relationships in families has traditionally been viewed as the woman's domain, the stepmother's self-esteem may drop. Feelings of guilt and loss of self-esteem reduce one's ability to be a good parent. This loss of self-esteem and esteem by others can lead to a woman trying harder, and failing more, and her efforts are seen as wicked if she tries to control children who refuse to be controlled, and ineffectual if she does not. These expectations come from men and women alike, who have been raised to see the woman's role chiefly as mother and nurturer. In a stepfamily, however, this expectation sets the woman up for failure.

Although stepmothers have the most difficult roles, and are viewed the most negatively (Ahrons and Wallisch, 1987; Visher and Visher, 1988), there are expectations of stepfathers which are problematic, too (Stern, 1978). There is a societal view, often espoused by women as well as men, that mothers are not capable of being strict enough disciplinarians, especially with boys, and that stepfathers should assume the role of "shaping up the kids." Unfortunately, this role is often expected of them by the mothers themselves, and even counselors have been known to encourage the stepfather to take charge of the discipline. One woman (not in this study) reported to me her belief that her second marriage may have succeeded if her counselor had not told her husband to be in charge of her teenage son. The man became tired of trying and failing, so he left. Women have functioned well as single parents; they should be viewed as competent in areas of child rearing unless proven otherwise in specific cases.

When mothers or fathers expect a new spouse to come in as a parent to their children, they unwittingly set up the new spouse for failure. Attempting to take on a disciplinary role too soon has been found to impede stepfamily integration (Brown, 1986; Dahl, Cowgill, and Asmundsson, 1987; Hetherington, Cox, and Cox, 1985; Visher and Visher, 1982, 1988). The stepchildren do not see a new stepparent as having the authority to discipline them, and that authority also may be undermined by a biological parent out of the home. It is difficult to discipline when the authority to do so is not sanctioned or accepted. In extreme situations, these attempts have led to a cycle of violence: the stepparent attempts to discipline a child, the child rebels, the stepparent tries harder, and the child rebels more, so physical punishment is used with increasing physical force as the child resists.

Clinicians and scholars in the field have often recommended that biological parents be in charge of their own children, especially at first. This plan involves the stepparent coming in as a spouse of a parent, not as a parent. Rules of the house need to be discussed and agreed upon by as many people as possible, but each parent is in charge of his or her own children. The stepparent is then free to develop his or her own relationships with the children, and may or may not eventually develop a relationship which involves disciplinary action. The main focus between stepparents and children should be on building trust and respect for each other, and that has to come first. The stepparent is often required to handle situations alone, but as long as the rules are made by the parent, and the majority of big problem situations are handled by the biological parent, then the stepparent can enforce the rules when alone with the children, as would any child-care person.

What do these 20 families say about discipline, and do their ideas match those of the experts? For the most part, the well-functioning stepfamilies do agree with the idea of stepparents going slowly in regard to discipline, and on the importance of developing relationships first. Overall, the suggestions from these parents support Stern's research (1978) that it takes about two years for a step-relationship to develop to the point where the stepparent can take on the role of disciplinarian. In fact, a few of these families recommend that when the children are older, the stepparent never should assume that role. In other situations, however, the stepparents took the disciplinary role sooner than that.

GOING SLOWLY

Arnold Allen is a particularly good example of going slowly, and developing a relationship first, before assuming a disciplinary role. He had known the children first as a neighbor, and had baby-sat them. There was some adjustment going from sitter to stepdad to dad (he is now adopting the children because the biological father is out of the picture). Alicia's sons have gone from calling him "Arnold," to calling him "Arnie-Dad," to calling him "Dad." This situation is the opposite of many families in that he believes his wife is too strict. She did not want him to discipline her boys at first, nor did she want his advice about discipline. Alicia said to him, "I can discipline them; please give them love instead." In the interview with this family, Arnold said, "that request from Alicia freed me to carry on as I believed best; I developed the role of teacher with the children. The term discipline comes from the word disciple, which means to teach. I feel that is the most important aspect of being a parent. I developed a special relationship with the boys as a teacher and mentor." He recommended that stepparents watch and learn the family rules and patterns before joining in on rule enforcement. He said, "it is so important to see how a family has been operating before you come in with your own ideas. I saw that their biological father had spanked them a lot, so I took to teaching as a form of guidance." Arnold is a gentle man and he usually talks out issues with the children. Now, after almost four years of marriage, he is a parent to these children in every way.

This idea of going slowly was reiterated by many of these families. When the children were young at the time of the marriage, many stepparents did gradually take on disciplinary functions, as did Arnold in the above story. One stepmother who took on some disciplinary tasks at the time of the marriage noted that she had lived with the family and developed a close relationship with the children before the marriage. She, too, had gone slowly, but her groundwork was laid before the marriage. Because she did not work outside of the home, she needed some authority with her stepchildren, and the fact that they were young allowed her to gain that authority more quickly. Early on, the father was in charge when he was at home, and it was his rule that they mind her when he was gone. There were a few grudges at first, but her husband backed her up, and the children accept her authority now. She did not try to replace the biological mother, which was important. The biological mother and grandmother take care of the children frequently, so the father's rule to his children is "mind everybody." The children also receive love from many sources.

In families where both parents brought children into the marriage, most noted that it was important for each parent to be in charge of his or her own children, especially at first. With younger children, it is possible for the stepparents to gradually move into a coparent role, but usually that does not work well when there are older children. In one such complex stepfamily, there were two factors which helped them to avoid discipline issues creating problems: the fact that they knew and liked each other's children before the marriage and the fact that they can all have fun together. Jokes and good humor prevail, and no issue seems to be too sacred not to joke about. They said that they went very slowly in integrating the discipline plan where both adults could enforce rules.

IMPORTANCE OF MEETINGS

In the Nolan family, with children from both parents living in the home, they discussed the usefulness of having rules and responsibilities spelled out very clearly. They have had regular family meetings from the start, where they did just that. It is agreed that the biological parent is in charge of her/his own offspring generally, but that when one is gone, whoever is home is in charge of the younger children. The mother in the family says that she will not discipline her husband's teenage children, except in the discussion of curfews and rules at the family meetings. Since she does not have children this age, she would not feel comfortable in that role with them. His teenage children agreed that they would not feel comfortable with her in that role, either. Luckily, the children are not discipline problems, so the issues that do arise are usually smaller issues such as not picking up personal items.

This family is a relatively newly formed stepfamily, and they are very aware of what works and what does not. The whole family was verbal in this interview. There was general agreement that the stepparent should come in slowly at first, and should never assume the disciplinary functions with older children. The nurturing and supportive functions can begin sooner, and even those should not be premature or forced. Family members discussed how chaotic things had been at first, and they agreed that the family meetings helped to provide the necessary structure for discussion and rule setting.

The importance of family meetings, stressed so strongly by the Nolans, was noted by other families, too. If the stepparents do not take on the disciplinary role at first, and maybe never with older children, how do they have any say at all in the household? One stepmother noted this dilemma. She said that when her husband's teenage boy came to live with them after a quarrel with his biological mother in another part of the country, they followed the adage of the father being in charge of his son. Since she was at home more than her husband, running a business out of her home, she felt "absolutely powerless." The situation lasted only one year, and the son is now an adult living on his own. If the situation had lasted longer, the stepmother said that an alternative plan would have been found.

Family meetings are a way of addressing this dilemma. The stepparents have a say in setting the house rules, even if they are not in charge of enforcing them, and the biological parents can use these sessions to back up their spouses' authority to enforce the rules in certain situations. Furthermore, the children usually respond better to house rules when they are included in the decisions about them. Family meetings are an opportunity for the children to express their ideas on the subject.

In one family, the father had been the rule maker and disciplinarian when he was a single parent with half-time custody of his daughter. When the stepmother came in, he was used to being in charge, but the stepmother had ideas of her own as well. They had family meetings on a regular basis so that her ideas could be expressed also. The father stayed in charge of most issues regarding his daughter, but the stepmother became more involved gradually, issue by issue. She enforced rules about making beds and practicing piano, which the father had not enforced, and he stayed in charge of everything else. During the first year, they talked about rules a lot, and these rules were set out very explicitly at family meetings. When the father continued to feel caught in the middle, he told his daughter and his wife to work out their own differences, and they did. Now the rules are clear, the stepmother has very gradually gained some authority, and they get along well as a family. They no longer need the family meetings on a regular basis.

In a situation where the father travels for his job a great deal, his new wife needs some authority. At family meetings, the rules are clearly spelled out, with both the husband and wife agreeing, and the children having input. The fact that the wife is more lenient than her husband and had a good relationship with his children before the marriage has helped this plan to work well.

BIOLOGICAL PARENT STAYS IN CHARGE

The Owen family, from the service group, underscores the importance of the stepparent not forcing discipline on older children. Oscar Owen said, "The worst mistake I ever made was to come in and try to discipline Oliver. I ended up in jail." Early in the relationship, he spanked his stepson, and was arrested for it. The charges were dropped when the stepson admitted that he deserved the spanking, and that it had not been a beating, but Oscar decided then that it was not his job to discipline his wife's son. After that, the boy's discipline was left with Olive, who had developed a close relationship with her son over the many years as a single mother. Oscar then took on the role of man friend, taking Oliver fishing and on other activities that they both enjoyed. At the time of my interview with this family, Oliver was emerging into adulthood, and he and his stepfather both agreed that they now have a good relationship, and are able to laugh about the arrest. Oscar was very firm in his suggestion that the stepparent not take on a disciplinary role too soon, and perhaps never.

Oscar Owen's idea that the biological parent should stay in charge of discipline when the children are teenagers was a sentiment expressed by many of these families. One stepfather noted that the rules and discipline of his teenage stepdaughter were clearly his wife's responsibility, not his: "I need to respect the mother/ daughter relationship and not interfere with it." This man has come into this family quite recently and his wife has a very close relationship with her daughter. He sees his main role with this girl as the husband to her mother. He maintains a cordial and respectful relationship with her, but not an emotionally close one. He feels that it would be inappropriate, for example, to show physical affection for his stepdaughter. It is interesting to note that the daughter sees her stepfather as having more authority in the family than he feels he has.

Although most of the families believed that it was better to have the biological parent in charge of the discipline with older children, this procedure varied from family to family. In one stepmother family, the father is mostly in charge, but he backs up his wife if she disciplines in his absence. In a stepfather family, it works well for the mother to stay in charge of her offspring, because she is more the "take charge" type while her husband is more "mellow." This arrangement has worked well for them because it matches their personalities and they respect each other's differences. They admitted that it could be difficult for some parents not to have authority. In another stepfather family which also hosts his children some of the time, the rules and enforcement were set out before the marriage. They decided that they did not want a different set of rules for each set of offspring. In general, it is better to have similar rules for the children in the home, and this may require compromise and discussion in family meetings. In rare situations, however, differences need to be accepted.

One of the families from the service group is a good example of accepting differences. In this complex stepfamily, discipline had been a major problem. The partners in the marital couple both handle conflict differently, and so do their children. The mother in this household tends to verbalize her anger, and her son knows this trait in her and waits for it to blow over, and in a short while they are fine again. His son, however, is not accustomed to open expression of anger, and he becomes quiet to avoid conflict, which frustrates the stepmother, because it seems resistant to her. This is a family in which various members clearly attach very different meanings to events. The wife's family views open expression of emotion as positive, and getting anger out as a healthy way of relieving tension. In the husband's family, however, open expression of anger is viewed as signifying serious problems, and to apologize and get beyond it is seen as avoidance of the basic underlying anger which needs to be resolved. This difference is so fundamental that it can not be resolved. For this family, the answer is for each to discipline his or her own child, and to accept that there are different rules for the children of the house. Things have gone better since they agreed to this plan.

SITUATIONS WHERE PARENTS ARE EQUALLY IN CHARGE

The Klein family has found that it has worked well for them to both be in charge of discipline. Both have been unemployed at different times, so it depends on who is home at the time. They believe that this plan has worked for them because her child was very young when the stepfather joined the family, and they had another mutual child soon. It seemed natural for the parents to share in discipline.

A family from the service group also found it to work well to have both parents discipline both sets of children, because the children are all very young, and the adults have similar ideas on discipline. Furthermore, this family is more marginal economically, and less time is spent on thinking about the meanings of people's behaviors; they pragmatically do what works.

SUMMARY

What common themes can one draw from these stories, if any? First, it is important to individualize; each family has to find its own unique way of operating. Beyond that, however, it usually works best if the stepparent does not come in as a disciplinarian right away. The recommendation from the Allen family, for the stepparent to join the family from the position of an outsider, noting the family's rules and patterns, and then to come in more as a teacher and mentor, and a backup to the parent, makes sense. Another general rule would be for the family to have meetings about rules of the house, especially at first. One family noted that they had regular meetings which had broken down during a move, and they have noticed the difference. While many families may find family meetings useful, they are especially important for stepfamilies.

Stepparents may more quickly become partners in raising the children when the children are younger, the noncustodial parent is either not very involved with the children or is very cooperative with the former spouse, and a firm relationship has formed between stepparents and children before the marriage. There does need to be a set plan for what the stepparent is or is not in charge of when the parent is gone. Again, clear expectations set in family meetings and even posted on the refrigerator seemed to help in this regard.

The last question to be asked is, "Was there a difference between these two groups of stepfamilies in this regard?" When these 20 families were charted on a continuum from stepparent disciplining as a parent to all discipline by biological parent only, the service families clustered between stepparent disciplining to midrange, and the high-functioning families had a wider range of patterns, but clustered more toward the end of biological parent only. When one considers the fact that the high-functioning families had been married longer, this finding seems to be more striking. The two guidelines heard most frequently from all of the families were "flexibility" and "clarity." Since the terms might be viewed as opposites by some, each family needs to find the balance between the two, recognizing the importance of both.

Chapter 4

Family Roles

Family roles have been defined by Epstein, Bishop, and Baldwin (1982, p.124) as "the repetitive patterns of behavior by which family members fulfill family functions." Epstein and associates have further outlined the necessary functions that are the basis for family roles as provision of resources, nurturance and support, adult sexual gratification, personal development, and maintenance and management of the family system. Role is a transactional concept; it is a set of behaviors which are based on expectations, obligations, and prescriptions which are expressed in a relationship. Further, these roles in families are tied to status or position in a family (Hartman and Laird, 1983).

Traditionally, the provision of resources has been viewed as the man's role, while nurturance and support have been the woman's role. Although these rigidly applied gender roles are no longer viewed as functional by many families today, and role flexibility is increasing in some families, these role expectations are especially maladaptive for most stepfamilies. As McGoldrick and Carter (1988) note, these traditional family gender roles have "no chance at all in a system where the children are strangers to the wife and where the finances include sources of income and expenditures that are not in the husband's power to generate or control" (p. 400).

Roles, then, are basically "who does what," and most family theoreticians agree that stepfamilies require some differences in this regard. A problem in redefining roles within a family system, however, is that these roles have been prescribed by the larger community system, and ingrained in the persons entering the family. Thus, a stepparent has expectations of her or himself, based on community expectations, which are part of that person's belief system developed over many years. Furthermore, those expectations continue to be reinforced by others in the community. For example, a school teacher who calls home with concern about a student is most likely to ask to speak to the woman in the family, even if she is not the biological parent.

In the last two decades, role strain has increased in most families as the role definitions become less clear, and as both parents take on more responsibilities. This strain is especially increased in stepfamilies, however, because the stepparent role is characterized by loss and gain of roles (Visher and Visher, 1979), there is lack of clarity regarding parenting roles and boundaries (Ahrons and Rodgers, 1987; Giles-Sims, 1984), and there is a lack of congruence between how stepparents think they should feel and act and how they in fact do (Whitsett and Land, 1992).

In a 1992 study of stepparents (Whitsett and Land, 1992), role strain is defined as those conflicts and challenges people encounter as they perform their roles. These researchers found stepparents to be more vulnerable to role strain than other parents, and that stepmothers reported more role strain than did stepfathers. They explained this finding by the fact that women are still expected to fill the primary nurturer and caretaker roles, and that even when these expectations are not overtly stated, societal forces and the woman's own expectations prescribe that role. They studied coping patterns in stepfamilies, and found that self-esteem of the stepparent and marital satisfaction of the married couple correlated positively with decreased role strain. A problem here, however, is that a lack of self-role congruence can lead to a loss of self-esteem, (that is, feelings of worth go down when people can not live up to their own expectations), and role strain can lead to decreased marital satisfaction. Although there may seem to be a hopeless circle here, these findings do suggest the importance of focusing on the marital relationship over parental roles in developing healthy stepfamilies. These investigators also found that the role strain decreases over time as couples are married longer, which can be a hopeful finding for stepfamilies, and which is consistent with the findings of my study with these 20 families. Last, Whitsett and Land's study pointed to the need for clarity regarding role expectations.

This question of role expectations in families overlaps with all of the other questions asked. For example, in the last chapter, the parental role of discipline was addressed, and it was noted that it is usually more useful if the stepparent does not try to come into the family as a parent, and especially not as a disciplinarian. In future chapters issues of money and relationships will be addressed, which certainly relate to role structure. It is difficult for most men to carry on the role of sole bread winner, for example, when there are several sets of families involved.

In the study of this question with these families, we asked what stepparents were called and how tasks were allocated among family members. In other words, who did what to manage and maintain the family system, how were those decisions made, and how clearly were the expectations stated?

WHAT TO CALL NEW FAMILY MEMBERS?

In the Foster family, good stepparent relationships were described by two teenage children. The 16-year-old daughter of Mr. Foster, in speaking about the relationship she has with her parents, said, "I feel close to Frances; she has been married to dad since I was a little girl. We are definitely a family. On the other hand, I also feel that my mom and her husband, Sam, are family. I feel like we (she and her brother) have two families, and that seems normal to us." Her brother agreed, and the two of them went on to describe how they move back and forth between their parents' homes every week, making the move at a prescribed time on Sunday evening. When I asked them what they called their stepmother, they looked surprised at the question and said, "Frances," as if there were no other options. Yet, there was an obvious closeness between these teenage children and their stepmother. This closeness was further demonstrated when the children discussed how they came to move every week. "At first we moved twice a week, and that was too confusing, and then we moved every two weeks, but that was too long, for whichever family we were with, we began to miss the other family. Every week is just right, and once we found this pattern to work, we just kept it." Another sign of closeness was when Flora and Frederick both talked of being a bit jealous of what their dad and stepmother did when they are gone. "We wonder what they are doing, and we think they are having fun and maybe don't miss us enough." While this statement was made as a joke, there seemed to be some real sentiments there, too.

They think of Frances as their stepmom, and Sam as their step-dad, but they feel love and respect for them both. They follow the rules of whichever house they are in, the "house rules." Luckily, the rules do not differ too much between the houses, but they say that if there were different rules, they would follow the rules of each house. They have bedrooms of their own in both homes, and they keep clothes and other personal objects at both places. They are expected to help with household chores at both houses, and those expectations are made clear. They belong to their father's church, and can get there from their mother's house, but they occasionally visit their mother's church. The mother and her husband moved into the same school district as the father, so the children could get to school from either place, but they are definitely not neighbors.

In this family, the stepmother works with her husband in making and enforcing the house rules. The children were young when Frances and Frank married, and they believe that is one reason why it has worked well for her to be involved in the discipline. The parents said that it also worked because the whole process of creating this stepfamily was very deliberate and carefully planned. Frank and Frances dated for six months before Frances met the children. He did not see any sense in the children meeting her until he was sure there was a real relationship, and she did not want to meet his children until she was sure Frank was marrying her because he loved her, not because he wanted a stepmother for his children. They then dated as a family for another year and a half. Frances developed a relationship with the children during that courtship period, and before the marriage they agreed on the fact that rule making and enforcement would be equally shared by Frances and Frank. Because the children were young and because they had gotten to know Frances well before the marriage, this plan worked. Although she is an equal partner with her husband in running the house and in raising the children, she has never tried to usurp the role of mother. There was no mandate for them to call her mother or to love her, just to respect her as their father's wife and co-head of the household. Over the years, however, that love and closeness have developed, partly because it followed its own course and was not prescribed.

What to call a stepparent is an important issue because it also suggests that person's role. If a parent says to a child, "this person is going to be your mom (or dad) now, so call her mother," that sets up a role expectation that this new adult in the house is going to replace another parent, and that this new person in the home should be loved and obeyed as a parent. Almost universally, these 20 families recommend against that approach (one of the service families was an exception). The terms mother and father seem to have very special meanings attached to them, and can not be applied to as many people as other terms can. The terms grandma and grandpa, for example, can apply to more people comfortably. Most of these children felt free calling stepgrandparents "grandma and grandpa" if they saw them frequently, and many enjoyed counting for me the number of aunts, uncles, and cousins they had from the many relationships. In fact, when those were supportive relationships, the children viewed the larger number of relatives as a source of comfort and pride, and they enjoyed describing these relatives in the interviews. For most of these children, however, the terms of mother and father seemed very special, and were not used with stepparents even when the relationships were close.

Most of these families found it useful for extended family members to negotiate what to be called with the children. For example, many reported that it worked well when a grandparent said something like, "You may call me grandma if you like, or you can call me Mary, or you may call me grandma Mary. What would you like?" These same families, however, did not report such negotiation around the parental terms. To suggest, "You can call me mom if you like" implies that would be the desired form, and most children reported needing to reserve that term for the real mother, whether she was close by, distant, or even deceased. It seems that one reason there can be more grandparents than parents is because of the implied roles inherent in the terms. For example, the grandparent role usually means nurturing and special times, and no child can get too much nurturing and special attention. On the other hand, the parental role usually carries a strong sense of obligation, responsibility, love, respect, authority, and power. It is more difficult to maintain that delicate relationship with many people.

The fact that most of these children called their stepparents by their first names indicated that they did not view them as a mom or dad, but that did not interfere with the development of good relationships. In fact, by not having a mandate to love and obey, the relationships could more easily flourish, and love often did develop. The stepparent role can be a very special one, allowing for different patterns to develop that are not based on prescribed roles.

As one stepfather said, "If stepparents try to set themselves up as equal parents, they set themselves up for failure." He is called by his first name, and aims to have a friendly relationship with his stepdaughter, but does not take on the parental role. There were some situations, however, where it did seem to work well for the stepparents to take on a stronger parental role, and in some situations they were called mom or dad. In two situations where this was true, the now adolescent children had lived with their stepfathers since they were very young, and in both families there was a mutual child (sibling to the adolescent) who reinforced the father term. Furthermore, in these two situations the mothers had full custody and these adolescents rarely saw their biological fathers. Furthermore, they noted, the term dad came gradually, and was not mandated.

In other situations where it did work to call the stepparent mom or dad, this practice also was taken on very gradually, and was usually begun by the child. In some situations, the child goes back and forth between first name and a parental term. In only two situations, one service and one high-functioning family, did this term begin at the time of the marriage. In one situation, the Allens, the stepfather had been a baby-sitter and had been very close to the children, and the biological father had been out of the picture for some time and not kept contact. Even then, the children themselves chose what to call him.

WHO DOES WHAT?

The Nolan family represents a complex family structure of his, hers, and theirs. They said that they tried several systems for chore responsibility before finding a plan that worked. They found the list of rotating chores too confusing, and they eventually decided to ask all family members to be in charge of their own chores (for example, making beds, picking up after themselves, putting their dishes in the dishwasher, doing their laundry) to the degree that they are able and old enough. Then whoever happens to be free when help is needed, such as setting the table, is asked to do that. Both spouses cook and shop. In this situation, both adults are professional people, and they are able to afford a daily housekeeper. For their large family, with children of many different ages, this plan seemed to work best.

In looking at roles within a household, I also asked: Who does what around the house? How is that decided? Who goes to whom for what? In this regard, our families reinforced the ideas suggested in the stepfamily literature (McGoldrick and Carter, 1988; Visher and Visher, 1988) that there needs to be more role flexibility in stepfamilies. In all but two of these families, one from each group, both parents were employed, and all but one of these employed persons were employed outside of the home (one was a day-care provider in her home). It is interesting that these families frequently not only had two bread winners, but the husbands' and wives' jobs were more equal than is often found in families. In the high-functioning families, for example, of the 12 families where the women worked out of the home (one was not employed and another woman ran a business out of her home), six of the couples had both partners at about equal-level positions, three had men in higher positions, and three had women in higher-level positions. In many situations, for example, both were professionals or both were in technical jobs. In the service families, two had both parents holding professional positions and two had both technical workers, one had the woman employed part time, and one had the woman not employed out of the home. In summary, these stepfamilies did not expect the man to be the sole provider for everybody's children, and there was more equality in sharing the task of supporting the family.

Similarly, in most of these families, and all of the high-functioning families, both adults in the home were engaged in household tasks. In some of the families, there were task divisions as to who does what, for the sake of clarity, but other families reported that "everybody does everything, whoever is here." The children were generally involved in household tasks too, and all members shared the work. Generally, it seemed to work best if there were some task divisions, if they were not held too rigidly. For example, in one high-functioning family, the woman was usually in charge of cooking and cleaning and the man was in charge of laundry and yard work. However, they flexibly shared chores, for example he would often pitch in with the cleaning, and she sometimes did laundry. In one family where the woman did stay home and take care of the children, and the man worked outside of the home, he said that he liked to clean the house when she was grocery shopping just to surprise her. In that family, there were several young children to manage, which is a full-time job in itself.

One family noted that they reversed the traditional roles in that she likes to do lawn work, and he likes to cook. In another family, the wife continued to do all of the housework as well as work outside of the home. She said that this was her choice, she had been a single parent for a long time, is used to being in charge of the home, and likes doing things her own way. There was some resentment about the children not helping enough, however, and this was one of the families seeking counseling. Several families found it worked best to have household chores for the children posted on the refrigerator. The importance of family meetings to discuss the household chores was also repeatedly emphasized.

SUMMARY

These families agreed with the literature on the subject (McGoldrick and Carter, 1988; Visher and Visher, 1988) that in stepfamilies it works best not to have the gender roles defined as clearly as with many families. In these families, both parents need to take on the nurturing and provision functions. As noted in the previous chapter, the discipline is usually best done by the biological parent, not the stepparent, especially as the family is first forming. In addition, the biological parent needs to be the main nurturer in the family. Parents who have lived alone with their children after a divorce or death of a spouse are usually very close to those children, and if the stepparent tries to intrude on that closeness, resentment is likely to occur. So, the nurturing and discipline roles are taken on according to who is the biological parent more than by gender. This creates a different structure from the one prescribed by some family therapists who advocate against cross-generational alliances (Minuchin, 1974). In these families, we saw a need for the parents to maintain a delicate balance between emphasizing their marriage relationship and allowing for the special relationship and ties between child and parent which may exclude the stepparent at times, both of which these families recommend. These issues will be discussed further in the chapter on relationships (Chapter 6).

Just as both partners need to be involved in child-rearing functions, usually both parents must be involved in generating income, too, especially if they bring children with them into the marriage. How money management works in these families will be discussed in the next chapter. When one part of the role structure changes, so do the other parts. Thus, when child rearing and income production become more equally shared, by necessity so do the other aspects of family life, such as household chores. In most of these families there was a high degree of role flexibility.

As discussed by Visher and Visher (1979), the stepparent role is often characterized by loss and gain of roles. The transition required here demands flexibility, but, as noted by Maglin and Schniedewind (1989), it can offer the opportunity for exciting and fulfilling new roles developed to meet personal needs, since there are not the prescribed societal roles. For example, a parent who does not have custody of the children after a divorce has lost the role of full-time parent and spouse. That parent can develop a very special relationship with the children, however, and it is often a more conscious and deliberate parenting effort. If that person then remarries, and acquires stepchildren, the opportunity for a very special and different relationship can develop where new rules can be made. If a stepparent role is viewed as different from a parent role, then this creative restructuring of new roles can be discussed and individualized around the needs and wants of those involved.

The role of spouse takes on special importance in these stepfamilies. A chief purpose of a first marriage is often to begin a family through procreation and to share in child rearing functions. In stepfamilies, however, the purpose of marriage is more often to support and nurture each other, not to be coparents in raising children. Thus, the spousal role needs special attention, and most of these families emphasized the importance of the marital couple having time together away from the children, and giving special energy to the relationship, while still allowing special parent-child relationships. This plan may involve more one-on-one time among family members, in addition to family activities.

Chapter 5

Money Management

Money management is closely related to role division, discussed in the previous chapter. Who earns the money (role of bread winner), who manages household finances (role of manager), and who allocates resources and makes the decisions (head of household) are important issues for most families. In second marriages these issues become further complicated by the involvement of more people and by different sources of income, and there are more questions as to who is entitled to what. In stepfamilies, there is usually a second marriage for at least one of the spouses. While this book is not about problems, as noted in the chapter on discipline, it is instructive for stepfamilies to see how potential problem areas have been handled by high-functioning stepfamilies.

Money management is the area in which there was the least agreement among the families in this study. It was also the area bringing the most concerns and disagreements, even in the high-functioning families. No other question stirred up so much controversy as did this question about money management. Money is often cited in the popular literature and in advice columns as a major source of family conflict in any family type, and most clinicians would agree that it is commonly cited by their clients as a source of disagreement. A surprising finding in my review of the literature on stepfamilies and on family therapy, therefore, was how infrequently the topic of money was discussed in the academic press. In this chapter, I will summarize the sparse literature on the subject, and then relate the stories of these 20 families, to see if their ideas back up the opinions expressed in the literature.

Guerin, Fay, Burden, and Kautto (1987), in their book on treating marital problems, cite money as a common source of marital conflict. They also note that money is a catchall organizing point for numerous other problems. They take the position that marital therapists need to be knowledgeable about financial matters and the relationship process that underlies them, in the same way that they need to be knowledgeable about human sexuality. As a family therapist, I strongly agree with that position. These authors offer four guidelines which they have found useful in assisting families to resolve financial problems, and I believe that they are especially useful in working with stepfamilies.

1. Money inherited or acquired by a person prior to marriage belongs to that person unless negotiated otherwise before the marriage.
2. Money earned by either spouse during the marriage belongs to both spouses unless negotiated otherwise prior to the marriage.
3. Money inherited during the course of a marriage belongs to the spouse who inherited it unless otherwise agreed upon at the time of the inheritance.
4. Children are the financial responsibility of the biological parents, even after divorce whenever possible, and even if one stepparent is quite wealthy. (p. 57)

They further note the importance of separating the financial realities from the relationship as much as possible.

McGoldrick and Carter (1988), in their discussion of differences of gender roles in stepfamilies, have noted that the idea that men should earn and manage the money can no longer work when some sources of income and expenditure are not in their power to generate and control (such as alimony, child support, earnings of ex-wife and current wife). Other authors have noted that money management may be especially problematic or complicated in stepfamilies (Goetting, 1982; Hartin, 1990; Knaub, Hanna, and Stinnett, 1984; Messinger, 1976). While the academic literature on money matters in stepfamilies is sparse, there is agreement among those who have written on the subject that money matters are especially complicated in stepfamilies, that symbolic issues regarding money need to be distinguished from real money issues, and that stepfamilies need different rules and norms from biologically based families for handling money matters.

A folk wisdom about money in families is that family integration and strength can be measured by the degree of sharing resources. The practice of sharing everything is often espoused as an ideal: "There is not his and hers but only ours." Attempts at following this maxim can produce problems in many situations, and may be especially problematic in stepfamilies, where one parent may be paying support for children elsewhere and the other may be receiving support for children in the home. In addition, grandparents may send money and gifts to some children, and other grandparents may send to others. One family may be used to the children having expensive lessons or memberships while the family that becomes part of them through remarriage may not believe in the importance of these special privileges. Some family members believe that teenage children should earn their own spending money while others believe in an allowance system instead. One parent may send out more in child support than the other parent receives in child support. As noted in letters to the editor of *Newsweek* (Letters, 1992), in response to an article on "Deadbeat Fathers," some fathers resent sending money to an ex-wife if they do not believe that the money is going to the children, but may be used by the mother or even her boyfriend. On the other hand, many women wrote to respond that their ex-husbands were living in luxury, ignoring their own children living in poverty. Today, more fathers are receiving custody of their children than in previous times, and the extent to which ex-wives are timely in support payments remains to be seen. What do the families interviewed here have to say about these issues?

As noted earlier, this subject brought out the most conflict within families, and it was also the subject which had the least agreement among families. This is an area in which each family's idiosyncratic nature is demonstrated; each needed a different plan to fit its own needs. Several families had tried different plans before they found one that seemed most satisfactory; others were still experimenting. Here, the families are grouped roughly into two categories: those who mostly pooled their resources and those who mostly kept the resources separate. Related money matters such as who is in charge of family accounting, allowances for children, and child support are also discussed.

KEEPING THE MONEY SEPARATE

The Wilson family from the service group is a good example of a family that keeps money separate. Mr. Wilson said that this plan is "the one thing that we have done right." In fact, he added that this plan has been "crucial" for their family functioning. He also expressed the idea that if they had worked out a similar plan for child raising to what they have for money management, they may have had fewer problems.

Mr. Wilson seemed proud of their financial plan; he said that this plan underscores that each partner is a person in his or her own right, not just an appendage of the other. In their family, each spouse has a separate account in which his or her salary is deposited, and then each pays into a joint account for household expenses such as mortgage payments, home repair, utilities, and home-owner's insurance (each pays his or her own auto payments and insurance out of the separate accounts). Any support he pays for his children (he has a 12-year-old son with him on a half-time basis who was there for the interview, and two adult children living on their own but still needing help) comes out of his account. He also handles his own credit card bills and personal expenses and his children's lessons and clothes. Mrs. Wilson's account contains her salary and the child support she receives for her son who lives in the home on a full-time basis. She pays for her son's clothes and allowance, her own credit card bills, and personal expenses out of her account. Mr. and Mrs. Wilson alternate buying the groceries out of their separate accounts.

While both partners in the Wilson marriage agree that this plan is a good one, and that separate accounts have been important for them, they disagree as to how well it works. While Mr. Wilson feels very good about it, Mrs. Wilson feels some irritation at times because she thinks he gives more money to his children than necessary. For one thing, he has three children and she has one child, and, furthermore, her son is not involved in the lessons and other activities that his son is. She says she sometimes resents so much of their money going to his children instead of to household expenses or couple activity. On the other hand, he says that this is how the money would be spent if they had not met and married.

In all, the families who kept their money separate were in the minority (seven: three from the service sample and four from the high-functioning group), but those that did believed that this plan was important for their functioning well. The families that did keep money separate generally followed the Wilson's plan of having a joint account as well as separate accounts. There was a continuum of how separate the money was kept. For example, the Davis family pooled most of their money, but was put into this category because the child support for her child was generally kept out to pay her daughter's bills. When no child support is received, however, the stepfather pays the bills for her. The Hall family, from the high-functioning group, also fell somewhat between the two groups and is moving now from separate to pooled, as the family has been together for many years. However, they were counted in the separate group because Hank's child support payments go directly to him for "shoes and school fees." Both parents pitch in to pay other bills as needed. Mr. Hall's income is larger but hers is more steady, so she tends to pay regular bills and he the special and larger ones. The Butterworth family in the pooled group is thinking that they need to separate their money more, and is moving in the other direction from the Halls. They believe that it is important for the boys' child support money to be kept separate for them, but they have not yet worked out a plan for doing so, so they were counted as "pooled."

Just how complicated money issues can be for these families is exemplified by the Davis family. They are a high-functioning family who kept money separately because, among other reasons, he pays out child support, she has a son in college, she receives child support, and she had debts when their marriage began. They maintain a total of seven separate accounts and one joint account, but are moving toward putting more into the pooled account and reducing the number of separate accounts. They hope to pool all of the money eventually.

POOLING ECONOMIC RESOURCES

On this continuum from separate to pooled money, a majority of the families (13: three from the service group and ten from the high-functioning group) were counted in the "mostly pool" category. There were not distinguishing characteristics between the families who pooled or shared money, rather each family has worked out a plan which works best for its individual situation, and, as noted above, many families moved back and forth between these plans.

Mrs. Ibsen stated her belief that "We're a family so we pool our resources." This belief was echoed by members of other families from this group who pooled resources. Mrs. Ibsen does not have children and her husband has two, a daughter in college and a son at home with him. His ex-wife does contribute some money for support of the boy, and she also helps the daughter with college expenses. The child-support money for the son, Ian, goes into a central pot of money, as do the salaries from both Mr. and Mrs. Ibsen. Mr. Ibsen's salary is larger than Mrs. Ibsen's, but hers is more steady and provides family benefits. Mr. Ibsen has a selling job that is rather new because his previous job was in his ex-father-in-law's company. That job ended with his first marriage.

In this family, Mrs. Ibsen handles all of the finances, as she likes to manage money. Since Mr. Ibsen travels a lot, this plan is helpful to him. The economic plan is simple: all of the bills are paid first, and if there is any money left they either buy or do something special. Each member of the family, including the children, receives a small allowance for personal spending which nobody questions. The college-age daughter holds a job to help with school expenses, to supplement the money she gets from her mother and from her father. She has a room in this family's home to come to on school vacations, which she appreciates since her mother shares an apartment with a roommate. Although Mrs. Ibsen writes the checks and distributes allowances, she and her husband discuss money issues and are in basic agreement. For them, this plan works well.

Although the Ibsen family did not seem to have problems with pooling money, as they have a good family income with basically enough to go around, what about a family with strained resources? Interestingly enough, pooling money was not a problem for the poorest family in this study, either, but was somewhat problematic for some families in the middle. The Peterson family lived on one income and was assisted by Aid To Dependent Children. This supplemental public support was necessary for Mrs. Peterson to raise her children because her husband's job did not pay well nor provide health benefits, three of four children were hers not his, and her ex-husband had left the state and does not pay child support. Three of the children were preschoolers and Mrs. Wilson stayed home to care for them. All of his salary and her benefits went into one pot which Mrs. Wilson carefully budgeted. Mr. Wilson's ex-wife was unable to send support money or care for her daughter because of a chronic illness. (An afternote here is that Mrs. Wilson did find a job and got off welfare two years after this interview, thanks to a work training program through the state which also provided day care.) This family had many economic problems just paying the bills, but they did not have arguments over money, and the pooling worked well for them, too.

Pooling money did not work so well for all of the families, however. The Taylor family, from the service group, pooled their resources, and yet money created many problems for them. Mrs. Taylor, who brought one child into the marriage, resents the money her husband spends on his two children who also are in this home. His children are older and he is planning on putting them through college (one leaves next year and one in two years). She worries that this money is coming out of their household account and that there will not be enough left to send her son to college when that time comes (he is only nine now). Her husband assures her that he will also help her son in college, but she does not trust him yet. This lack of trust is probably due in part to the fact that this couple has only been married 1 1/2 years, that he has been married twice before, and because she feels that his children spend money foolishly and do not budget. She and her husband have quite different views about money habits, and this issue has brought about many arguments, and has led her and her son into therapy. Perhaps for them, separating out some of the money would have been useful, but that still may not have solved the problem.

In another of the service families, the Smiths, money created a problem, but their problem did not relate to their pooling resources. The problem for them was that both of them resented the money he paid to his ex-wife in child support because the money did not seem to go for the children, and they suspected it went for the mother's drugs. They were also annoyed that her ex-husband did not pay support for her two children who lived with her and Mr. Smith. They pooled the resources they had, and both have good incomes, but they both felt resentful about their ex-spouses. If anything, this resentment seemed to draw them closer together, and pooling money was not a problem.

An ex-spouse also causes resentment over money for the Lange family. Her sons' biological father has had almost no contact with the children since he remarried, nor does he send support money for them. When the biological father does send any money, he sends a check directly to the boys, which angers Mrs. Lange, since this family has the pattern of pooling the money. Her sons have turned the checks over to her for the family pool, however, so the problems are not within this unit, but with anger at her ex, and some guilt that her husband has to help her support her children.

The Martin family is an example of a family who believed that they should keep money separate when they first married, but they never got around to organizing the plan. Now, two years after the marriage, they have found that pooling their money has worked well. Several other families similarly expressed that they believed in separating money, but just found it more expedient to pool it. The Martins said that their plan is a simple one; the salaries go into a single account and checks are written on that account. The only child in the home is hers, and Mr. Martin makes considerably more money than does Mrs. Martin, but he feels no resentment, and is happy to have this family as his own. The daughter earns some money tutoring other children and contributes some of her income into the household pot, saving some for her personal use.

SUMMARY

There does not seem to be a right way to handle money; each of these families needed to work out an individual plan. When it works, pooling money is easier and more of these families did that, but those families who kept money separately felt that it was important that they did so. While for this analysis these families were divided into two groups, those who pooled their resources and those who divided them, within those groups there were many different ways of managing money. For example, sometimes child support went into a general account and sometimes it was earmarked for the child, sometimes the husband paid the bills and managed the accounting, sometimes the wife did those tasks, sometimes these tasks were split with each partner paying her or his expenses, and still at other times the tasks were shared with both taking turns. Sometimes children were paid allowances, sometimes they were expected to earn their money, and sometimes they just asked for money needed. One common theme found in most of these families was that there was not one head of household economically; money matters were discussed and plans agreed upon by both of the marital partners as a team. While this is probably a good plan for most families, it seems especially important for stepfamilies because the economics are more complicated and decision making needs to be more egalitarian because of the divided loyalties.

No clear patterns were found to differentiate between those families who pooled and those who separated their money. There were not sharp differences by whether they were in the service or high-functioning group, by family structure, or even by length of marriage. In fact, two high-functioning families with similar structures fell into each of the groups, pooled and separate. In both the Foster family and the Jones family, the wives were professional women who had no biological children, and their husbands' children moved back and forth from their mothers' houses every week. Yet, the Fosters pooled their resources more, and the Joneses kept separate accounts, and both situations seemed to work well for them. With the Fosters, they pooled their money, kept a house with bedrooms for the children, and paid for the children's expenses during the weeks they were there. The children even had clothes and toys in each house which stayed there. The Fosters paid half of the children's school expenses, lessons, and camp from their joint account, and the biological mother and her husband paid the other half. In the Jones family, each professional partner kept his or her salary in separate checking accounts. He paid his child's expenses, including support to his ex-wife who had custody half-time, and his own expenses out of his account, she paid her expenses out of her account, and they shared household expenses. Mrs. Jones did buy things for her stepdaughter out of her account, but it was because she wanted to, not because it was expected. She believed that it helped her to bond with her stepdaughter to take her shopping with money from her own account.

While money was one of the least addressed topics in the academic literature, it proved to be one of the most interesting topics discussed with these families. It was clearly the topic that caused the most controversy and resentment within these families and the topic which had the least agreement between families. In this chapter, a wide range of money management plans have been discussed, and the ones found most useful have been highlighted.

Chapter 6

Managing Relationships

Relationship management is a central task in any family, but there are more relationships to manage, and often more problematic ones, in stepfamilies. The subject of this chapter underlies all of the other chapters, since everything else that occurs in families depends on the relationships between the members. Relationships outside the household are important, too, because when a stepfamily is first formed the network support is often low and the extended family relationships often strained (Whiteside, 1982). In this chapter relationships within families, relationships with ex-spouses and their families, and relationships with extended family and the social network are all addressed.

As noted by Visher and Visher (1988), the subgroups of coalitions and alliances within families are usually held together by loyalty to the larger family unit, but within new stepfamilies there are built-in alliances and coalitions without the overriding loyalty to the unit at large. A task for developing healthy stepfamilies is to create a sense of a family unit and loyalty to that unit. The development of a strong marital system without children feeling replaced, the development of stepparent-stepchild relationships without children feeling disloyal to their biological parents, and the development of relationships between children who are not related to each other and who may be giving up a favored sibling position (for example, oldest, youngest) are all central parts of this developmental task. Attention to who feels included or left out, to personal boundaries, and to physical space are issues which need to be addressed here. The potential for sexual attraction in stepfamilies must be faced, too, since the incest taboo is not as strong in stepfamilies (Robinson, 1984). That attraction can be between stepparent and child or between stepsiblings.

Even though it is important for stepfamilies to develop a sense of family, where members feel a part of the unit, the boundaries need to be permeable enough for children to move back and forth between households. Ahrons (1979) has conceptualized the "binuclear family," where children are raised in two interacting households. There is considerable evidence that children adjust better after divorce if they are able to maintain contact with both parents and with other relatives (Ahrons, 1981; Hetherington, 1979; Wallerstein and Kelly, 1980). There is even evidence that children form better relationships with stepparents when they are not cut off from the noncustodial parent (Furstenberg and Nord, 1985), although Clingempeel and Segal (1986) found that stepdaughters formed better relationships with stepmothers if their contact with the biological mother was limited. The importance of parents maintaining a civil relationship with each other after a divorce has also been discussed in the literature (Visher and Visher, 1988). When parents continue to quarrel, they have not psychologically separated from each other (Wallerstein and Kelly, 1980), which hinders the development of the stepfamily unit. An important task for developing stepfamilies, then, is to have a clear plan for allowing the children to continue visits and relationships with both biological parents and with grandparents and other relatives.

It is also important for the stepfamily's development to have support for the new unit from the couple's extended families and from other social networks. If a couple loses the support of friends, members of their church or other community organizations, or their own families, the integration of the new unit is much more difficult. In this chapter, we will look at how these families managed these relationship issues.

RELATIONSHIPS WITHIN FAMILIES

In asking questions about what was useful in developing relationships within these families, three basic themes emerged. First, was the rule to "go slowly." Second, was the emphasis on privacy and space, arranging as much personal space as possible. Third, was the importance of the marital relationship to set the foundation for everything else.

The injunction to go slowly overlaps with the discussion in the chapters on discipline and on roles (Chapters 3 and 4). Most of these families agreed that it works best not to push relationship development between stepparents and children and between step-siblings. In the discussion on discipline, the Allen family was used as a good example of going slowly; Mr. Allen slowly developed a good relationship with the children before taking on a parental role. He also recommended careful observation of the family rules before jumping into the relationship, and not forcing the relationship on the children. The Foster family is another good example of going slowly; the couple dated for over a year and a half, first alone and then with the children, before marriage. The Evans family had a similar story; Mrs. Evans did not expect her stepson to love her, she felt love had to be earned. She and her stepson began the relationship treating each other respectfully and they carefully scheduled time for him to be alone with his father, for couple time between Mr. and Mrs. Evans, and for family activity involving all three. Then she and her stepson began to plan activities together that were structured, such as her helping him with piano practice.

This careful structure is important to make sure all members receive some time with the people important to them. Visher and Visher (1988) have discussed how children can feel displaced when their parent remarries, because they had become the parent's confidant and buddy after the divorce, while living as a single-parent family. Care needs to be taken not to take away the special relationship, but to gradually build in the marital relationship as paramount. It is a delicate balance. Mr. and Mrs. Evans, for example, said that Emil still gets jealous when they go out as a couple without him. They are careful to give Emil time alone with each of them as well as family time, but have gradually built in more couple time and are holding to it firmly.

In the Davis family, Mrs. Davis and her daughter, Debbie, have a very close relationship, and Debbie is not as close to her stepfather, who is relatively new in the home. Mr. Davis is very careful to respect that relationship between mother and daughter, and works at not interfering with it. He does not hug or kiss Debbie, because he thinks it would be inappropriate, and because he does not want to be intrusive. Mr. Davis does, however, take Debbie fishing on occasion. This is an example of what was found in most families; special activities between stepparents and stepchildren were found to be important for relationship development. Where the stepparent and child are the same sex, special activities are especially healing, since those are usually the most difficult relationships in stepfamilies. Children often went to a stepparent over a parent on matters of special expertise, too. Having a skill to teach a child was found useful for many of these stepparents.

An example of going too quickly was cited by one of Mr. Nolan's sons. Mr. Nolan had already gone through a great deal of his grieving during the time his wife was slowly dying. Thus, he felt ready to remarry rather quickly, especially since his wife had requested that he do so. The new Mrs. Nolan had been a family friend, and they were surprised that the children reacted to their marriage so strongly at first. Things were just beginning to settle down at the time of the interview, two years later. In this interview, as the adults puzzled about the children's reactions, one of his young sons said, "It was just too soon, dad, it was just too soon." A strong marriage, a mutual child, and time have worked to this family's advantage; they now see themselves as very high-functioning, and indeed do appear so.

Several of the families emphasized the strong marriage as the foundation on which to build the stepfamily. Mrs. Nolan said that was what got them through the first two years. While it is important for the marriage to be strong, a good marriage does not ensure stepfamily satisfaction or contentment among the children (Clingempeel, Brand, and Ievoli, 1984; White and Booth, 1985).

Personal and physical space is an important issue in developing relationships in stepfamilies. When the families are formed, children often find themselves living with strangers. Having a space to themselves helps children not feel pressured to be close too soon. Many of these children spoke about the need to get away and be alone at times. Furthermore, since there may be sexual tensions that are not as prevalent in biologically based homes, it is important that special care be taken to ensure privacy for all family members and to have a more conservative manner of dress around the house.

The families interviewed for this project had all paid attention to the issue of space. When possible, each child should have his or her own room, or share with a same-sex blood sibling. Such a plan is not always economically feasible, however, especially for those children who visit as noncustodial children. All of these families spoke of moving for more space, adding on to an existing house, fixing up the basement, or putting dividers in existing rooms. As one father said, "Do whatever you have to, but make sure everyone has a space of his own."

The Foster family has an ideal arrangement in this regard. Flora and Frederick have their own rooms in both of the two houses that they move to and from every week. They keep clothes, toys, and books at both houses and do not even pack suitcases when they move. Very few families can afford that kind of space, however. The Davis family has a room for Debbie, who lives there on a full-time basis, but there is a boys' room in the basement for when his son or her son visits, and if they visit at the same time they have to share a room. Most of these families (ten of the high functioning and four of the service) moved when they got married or shortly afterward, not only for more space, but also to begin as a new family in neutral territory. Those that did not move had generally rearranged the house.

RELATIONSHIPS WITH EX-SPOUSES AND THEIR FAMILIES

After money management, relationships with ex-spouses came in second as a major source of conflict and contention. While there is not one way for these situations to be handled, for each family has different needs and issues, all of the families agreed on one thing: the importance of cooperation between parents and the importance of not getting the children caught in the middle of disputes. Not all of these families were able to practice what they believed best, however, and as with rituals discussed in the next chapter, they usually blamed their ex-spouses or families for the problems.

This is one area where there were clear differences between the service and high-functioning groups. In the high-functioning group, ten families had varying degrees of cooperation with their ex-spouses and their families, none had continual battles, in three families there had been a gradual decrease of activity with the parent to little or nothing, and in one there was a discontinued relationship. In the service families, only one had a cooperative relationship, three had conflictual relationships, two had lost contact, but none had a sudden cut-off. These were not clear-cut categories, because some families had some conflict but still cooperated, and others had some relationships severed or conflictual, while some remained cooperative. Still, 71 percent of the high-functioning families had basically cooperative relationships with ex-spouses, whereas only 16 percent of the service families did. Although there were several patterns that worked in the cooperative families, the common themes that emerged as helpful were having arrangements clearly spelled out and adhered to as much as possible, keeping conversations with the ex-spouse focused on the children, and having a civil but not a friendship relationship with the ex-spouse. The idea that it is preferable to continue friendships and chummy relationships between ex-spouses was not borne out in this study.

Several researchers in the field have discussed the importance of children maintaining contact with both parents following a divorce, except in special circumstances (Ahrons, 1981; Hetherington, 1979; Wallerstein and Kelly, 1980). One of these high-functioning families is an example of the negative effects of a total and sudden emotional cut-off. Mrs. Lange's sons, Larry and Lance, were cut-off from their father after his remarriage, and Mrs. Lange discussed this situation in the interview. Mrs. Lange and her first husband divorced about 11 years ago, when the children were preschoolers, and Mrs. Lange remarried two years later. The children's father lived in another state, but paid child support and maintained contact with the boys quite regularly at first. They visited him in the summer, and several times during the year. When he began to court another woman, she treated the children as special, and they thought that she liked them. The woman was very friendly to the boys until the time of the marriage, and then there was a total and sudden cut-off. For the last five years, the boys have had no contact from their father and no child support has been paid. This was one situation where I thought that the mother's negative discussion of her ex-husband's behavior was appropriate in front of the children, because it clearly took the blame off them. Apparently, the boys had been upset at first, and felt that they had done something wrong.

Mrs. Lange believes that the new wife just did not want the responsibility of being a stepparent, and that the children's father was not strong enough to stand up for what he wanted. Lance and Larry were pretty quiet as she spoke, but did not disagree with what she said. When I asked their opinions, they nodded and agreed with their mother but were embarrassed by the discussion.

The Langes know that cooperation can work, because Mr. Lange has children, now grown, from two previous marriages, and he and both ex-wives have cooperated for the children even when they were not on the best terms themselves. In addition, Mrs. Lange knows the role of stepmother herself, and can not understand why her boys' stepmother has shunned that responsibility. She is grateful that her husband is willing to be a father to her boys in every way, even financially, when that was not part of the bargain at the time of their marriage. (It should be noted, however, that Mrs. Lange has a well-paying job, also.) He has a good relationship with the boys, and tries to be extra supportive to them. One of his daughters is a college student who lives in the house part time. She and the boys get along well and consider themselves to be siblings.

The emphasis of this study is on healthy family functioning, and what seems to work. It is interesting, therefore, to note that in most of these families the children do maintain contact with the noncustodial parent and with grandparents and other relatives from that parent. In a random sample of divorced couples, 75 percent of the children had no contact with their fathers (Furstenberg and Nord, 1985), whereas in this study of healthy stepfamilies, 70 percent of the children have contact with the noncustodial parent. This figure is based on all 20 families, combining the service and nonservice groups, further demonstrating the point that all of these families are relatively well functioning. Of those families where there is little or no contact with the noncustodial parent, only one (the Langes, discussed above) experienced a total cut-off, and that involved only one branch of the family (her children, not his). In the other situations, there is one family in which there was a gradual decrease in visits over many years as a stepparent came in when the child was young. In two other cases, the mothers gave birth at a young age (one had a brief marriage, the other was not married), and the children were very young when the stepfather came into the picture, assuming the father role. In one case, the father was barred from visitation by the court, but the paternal grandparents have continued contact, even though the children have been adopted by the stepfather. In a similar situation, one mother has visitation limited by the court due to severe mental illness, but the maternal grandparents have continued contact.

In the remainder of the families, where there is contact, there is great variety as to the frequency of the visits, the arrangements, and the degree to which the relationships between the cooperating adults are cordial or conflictual. In fact, the term "visitation" may be wrong. As eight-year-old Emil Evans said, "I don't visit my mother; I live with her in the summer and I live with my dad during the school year." Frederick and Flora Foster expressed similar sentiments when they said, "We have two homes." Three families had arrangements where the children exchanged homes every other week; in two of those families, the Fosters and the Joneses, there was a very regular and planned pattern. In the Wilson family, just one of the children in the home (his, not hers) exchanged every week, and it was a bit looser and left to William to negotiate himself. With the Joneses and Fosters, an interesting difference was noted regarding how close they live to their ex-spouses for the convenience of the children (which was not an issue with the Wilsons because they live in a smaller town). For the convenience of the children, Mr. Foster's ex-wife and her husband moved into the same school district in which Mr. Foster lives and because it is considered a better school. They do not live close enough to be neighbors, however. The Jones family lives in the same block as his ex-wife for the convenience of Jessie. While it is convenient for Jessie to be able to go back and forth between the houses, there is not the distinct boundary as to where to be when, and as to who is in charge. The Foster's plan seems to have worked better than the Joneses'; being too close can bring about lack of privacy and some bad feelings. The clarity of the Foster's plan seems to be most successful.

In general, in the families where the noncustodial parent lives nearby, the children visit on occasional weekends, often every other weekend. Holidays and celebrations are shared; these arrangements are discussed in the next chapter. In families where one parent lives several states away, there is a larger block of time in the summer when the children visit, and often there is a holiday visit, too. Most of these families allow children to visit grandparents from the other parent's side, if they had a good relationship prior to the divorce. In some situations, the parents themselves had good relationships with their former in-laws, which they have maintained.

Conflictual relationships, when they occurred, were a source of stress for everyone involved. In the Smith family, from the service group, a main stressor was the ex-spouses on both sides. Mrs. Smith's ex-husband does not pay child support regularly, and is irregular in visiting the children. Mr. Smith's ex-wife causes even more problems in that she lives a lifestyle which the Smiths believe is detrimental to the children who live with her. The ex-wife discourages the children from visiting the Smiths, and she says negative things about them. The Smiths are concerned about her drug use and worried that she spends the child-support money on illegal activities. His ex-wife has told his children that his stepchildren have replaced them in his life. Mr. and Mrs. Smith handle the situation by having the children with them when they can, by trying to demonstrate that they care about his children, by modeling a different lifestyle, and then by recognizing that there are things out of their control that they have to accept. The Smith family also uses humor and fun together to alleviate the stress. The interview with the four of them was fun. The humor was not used as denial or sarcasm, but as tension relief from recognized problems.

SOCIAL NETWORKS

A great deal has been written about social networks, but suffice it to say here that involvement in extrafamilial social networks are beneficial for both individuals and families, diminishing the effects of stress and isolation (McCubbin et al., 1981; Ihinger-Tallman and Pasley, 1986). Ihinger-Tallman and Pasley cite several studies demonstrating the disruptive effects of divorce on social involvement, and they studied the effects of remarriage on that involvement. They note that remarried families may continue to be isolated because of the noninstitutionalized status of stepfamilies. If the family is cut-off from extended family because of the divorce, the situation is made worse. They found that the presence of children and a higher level of education correlated positively with integration into the community (1986). There is agreement in the literature that the presence of support networks is associated with stepfamily success.

The stories from these families do emphasize the importance of support networks in developing healthy stepfamilies. When these 20 families were put on a continuum from weak to strong social support and involvement, 13 of the 14 high-functioning families fell at the very strong end of the continuum, with one at the weak end. Conversely, five of the six service families fell at the weak end, with one at the strong end.

The Butterworth family is an example of a high-functioning family with many stressors and a very strong social support network which, they say, "has been essential." They have two sons by his first marriage and a daughter together. This is a situation where all of the extended family members have rallied to help with the care of a seriously ill boy, Ben, age five. Mr. Butterworth's ex-wife and her mother, and Mrs. Butterworth's own stepmother and her brothers and sisters all work cooperatively to help the Butterworths care for the boy. Mr. Butterworth's own parents are deceased. He is still close to his ex-mother-in-law, who is very supportive, and who has baby-sat all of the children at times, even the daughter by the new marriage. In addition to the strong extended-family support, there is very strong support from his church, which Mrs. Butterworth has joined. Not only do they receive support from the members of the church, they are active members who give back in time and effort to the extent that they can. Mr. Butterworth is also active in Little League with his older son, Bob, age nine.

The families at the high end of the social support continuum were connected strongly with at least two networks outside of the nuclear family; most had three or more. The support systems named most frequently were extended family, church, a close group of friends or professional associates, and involvement in community activities, often related to the children's school or sports activities. The social networks involve reciprocity: the families not only were supported by others, but they contributed and gave back. These reciprocal relationships with social networks help families become integrated into, and accepted by, the larger community.

The families discussed the importance of these connections; several said they have gotten through the difficult years with the help of friends, relatives, and often church members and clergy. Members of the two families where there was not extended family nearby talked about how their close group of friends served as extended family for them. In two families, the new stepmothers gave their own parents the opportunity to be grandparents for the first time. They talked about how the stepchildren served to bring them even closer to their own families and to related activities.

SUMMARY

The topic of relationships in stepfamilies has been studied and discussed in the literature a great deal (for example see, Ahrons and Wallisch, 1987; Clingempeel, Brand, and Ievoli, 1984; Clingempeel and Segal, 1986; Ihinger-Tallman and Pasley, 1986; Kurdek, 1989; Orleans, Palisi, and Caddell, 1989; Robinson, 1984). In this chapter, what was learned from these families regarding relationship issues in three areas has been explored. First, the area of relationships within the family unit was addressed, and the importance of not forcing parental roles or sibling roles too quickly was noted, as was the need for children to continue special relationships with parents. Second, the ways in which these families negotiated relationships with their ex-spouses and ex-in-laws for the sake of the children were noted and discussed. Last, the importance of support networks and of the family's integration into the community were addressed and examples of those supports for these families were noted.

transition
confirmation
wedding

healing

?

birthday (cake for breakfast)
graduation

identity - redefinition
adoption
Bar mitzvah

Chapter 7

Family Rituals and Traditions

Family theorists and therapists have borrowed the concept of rituals from anthropologists as a way of understanding the culture of families. As Hartman and Laird (1983) have stated, "if rituals stand at the very core of culture, since families develop their own cultures and are among the most central of transmitters of larger cultural processes, it may be that rituals also stand at the very core of family life" (p.106). While there has been considerable deliberation about the exact definition of ritual (Hartman and Laird, 1983; Roberts, 1988), for purposes of this discussion I will use the term to denote those behaviors which are prescribed, ordered, repeated, and have symbolic meaning.

Rituals provide a valuable function in family life by marking life-cycle changes, such as weddings, funerals, and birth ceremonies, by connecting families to previous generations, by providing mechanisms for resolving conflicts, and by linking individuals, families, and communities (Imber-Black, 1988). Rituals also provide a safe and manageable context for expressions of strong emotions, since time and space boundaries are made clear, and they foster a sense of identity for individual family members (Fiese, 1992). They can be especially important in stepfamilies, as they can reduce anxiety about change, demarcate boundaries and family roles, and connect families to the larger community. Rituals can make new relationship options available. Imber-Black (1988), in a discussion of rituals in family life, describes transition rituals, healing rituals, and identity-redefinition rituals. All three are important in stepfamilies. The formation of a stepfamily is a major critical incident in the life cycle because it disrupts (changes) the functioning of two family systems. It is an event which usually sends "ripples'' throughout the extended family system (Whiteside, 1982). A ritual around the joining together of these two units can facilitate that process of change. The healing rituals are important because the stepfamily members have had to deal with major losses as well as change (Visher and Visher, 1988). The identity rituals are important because so many roles have been interrupted and need redefinition: a son is now a stepson as well, mom's boyfriend is now stepdad, and the rules about who relates to whom and how are different.

In family life there are rituals to mark special occasions (such as graduations and weddings), there are rituals around special holidays (such as the celebration of Christmas or Chanukah), and there are everyday rituals (such as family prayers, bedtime stories, and meals together). Since the members of stepfamilies have developed certain patterns and traditions in previous family life, and have certain beliefs about the right way to do things, it is important to these new family units that some former traditions and rituals are kept from both sides to decrease the sense of loss and increase the sense of familiarity, and that new rituals and traditions are developed to mark this new unit as a family. Indeed, the creation of these rituals does help the new family unit develop its sense of being a family, as well as mark that boundary to others. These rituals can also help the new unit to become incorporated into the extended families and into the community at large.

In this chapter, family traditions are discussed as well as rituals, and sometimes the terms are used almost interchangeably. Traditions are ''the handing down of beliefs and customs from one generation to another, especially without writing'' (*Oxford American Dictionary*, 1980, p. 728). The key distinction is that a ritual involves a behavior that is repeated, usually with symbolic meaning, while a tradition is a belief or idea held over time. In family life, however, these two blend in closely, almost on a continuum.

For example, in the musical ''Fiddler on The Roof,'' the father sings about the importance of tradition. In that case, the custom of having the father choose a husband for his daughter is the tradition, but the wedding ceremony itself would be the ritual. In these stepfamilies, having sit-down dinners together may be a tradition, but when those meals are a time when the family has prayers together, and when there are certain prescribed behaviors, such as "this is when we all share our day's activities," then it becomes a ritual, too. In this discussion, the distinction between the two is not as important as assessing how rituals and traditions work together to help stepfamilies develop a stronger sense of family.

In these families, as in families in general, there is variation in the degree of ritualization. In this chapter, the ways in which these families celebrate life-cycle events, special holidays, and everyday occurrences are described, and the ways these rituals serve to facilitate change, heal, and bind the new family together are discussed.

LIFE-CYCLE TRANSITIONS

A major ritual for stepfamilies to mark their own beginning is the wedding itself. All of these families had a ceremony to which families and friends were invited and in most cases the children were involved, too, often as part of the ceremony. While there were ceremonies and receptions, they were usually smaller than in first weddings. In some situations, we (the graduate student who videotaped the sessions and myself) were shown the wedding pictures. Whiteside (1982), in her discussion of developmental processes in stepfamilies, notes the importance of the wedding in marking the transition and in helping the children and other family members recognize the permanence of the union. It stirs up residual issues of conflict in many parties, and it serves to reduce the children's fantasies about the parents' reunion. Even though the event may strain relationships in several areas, it is important for boundary marking. Furthermore, as noted by Roberts (1988), rituals serve to incorporate both sides of a contradiction. A wedding ceremony has within it both loss and joy, marking both endings and beginnings. The ceremony provides for the support and containment of strong emotions on both sides of the issue.

In addition to having had rituals around their own weddings, a few of these families have already had other life-cycle events to mark, such as weddings and graduations of the children. These events can also arouse conflict, such as who is invited to the party, and who sponsors the events. Several of these families expressed the view that for the children's special events, such as graduation or marriage, the biological parents should cooperate and keep their own roles as parents and the stepparents should attend in the role of spouse of the parent and stepparent to the child. There was also agreement that the extended families on all sides should be included. The guiding principle that this day is for the daughter or son, and the parental conflicts should be put aside for the day, was subscribed to by these families. However, in practice it did not always work that way for these families. From their perspective, the ex-spouses or their families got in the way of cooperation. In one situation, the ex-in-laws refused to attend a graduation party if the father and stepmother attended. This family decided not to make an issue of it. They did not attend the party, but they did attend the ceremony and had a small party for his daughter at a different time. Since they had custody, and more time with his daughter all along, they decided not to upset the girl at this important time. In these high-functioning families, this kind of sacrifice for the larger cause was not uncommon. As one parent said, "Keep your eye on the big picture."

HOLIDAY TRADITIONS

Most of these families saw the need to have special traditions and holiday celebrations to help them bond together. Most also recognized the need for flexibility about holidays, since there were several sets of relatives who wanted the children for these special days. There was a great deal of cooperation and compromise on the part of these families to make the holidays work, and they often had to give up previous ideas as to what to do when. In return, most of them had found ways to celebrate these holidays in satisfying and meaningful ways and still allow the children to visit other parents or grandparents. Some of the children in this study counted two or three Christmases or birthdays a year. Most of the families interviewed talked about the importance of special plans, and nine of these families, six high functioning and three from the service group, told specific stories about holiday cooperation involving either multiple holidays for the children or alternating by the year or the holiday. Some pretty complicated schemes were described.

The Jones family is a good example of how cooperation and

flexibility are important in making holidays work. Their situation and plan is typical of several that were described to me. The Jones family splits Christmas, Easter, and Jessie's birthday with Jessie's mother. Since they live near each other, Jessie spends part of each holiday with both families. Her mother thinks that it is her job to host the children's birthday party each year, so the Joneses have a small gathering of adult friends and relatives to celebrate the birthday. Jessie spends Christmas eve and Christmas morning with her mother, and has Christmas day, including the big dinner, with her father and stepmother. Mr. and Mrs. Jones have a big Christmas party for their friends every year, so they like having Jessie there for that.

They also have a big party on the Fourth of July, with a large picnic for their friends' families as the other big "tradition" they have begun. To ensure that they can have Jessie home every year for this big event, they have traded Thanksgiving, which is entirely the mother's. So, of five big holidays a year, three are shared and two are traded.

Mr. Jones brought in a birthday custom from his first marriage, and has declared having "custody of the custom." This tradition involves having a person dress up as a "birthday pig" and deliver presents in a Santa manner. This family is highly ritualized. They also celebrate half birthdays by having half a cake, half a card, and by singing half the song. They like to recognize events, and they celebrate most events by making and flying banners. Any awards or achievements earned by any family member is celebrated by the making of special banners and by having a family ceremony. The Jones family has lots of fun with special events, and it was enjoyable to hear them described. Their stories demonstrate how traditions, such as having birthday parties, can become rituals, with the banners, cakes, cards, and singing.

While not all of the families were as highly ritualized as the Joneses, many had holiday arrangements just as fixed and just as complicated. Most of these families believed that careful plans, no matter how complicated, made things easier. In the Taylor family from the service group, his two children want to spend Christmas with their mother so this family celebrates Christmas as a family unit early. Then, Mr. and Mrs. Taylor and her daughter get together with her side of the family for Christmas day.

In the Lange family, there is careful planning to involve everyone, even though her children do not see their dad anymore. They have one big Christmas celebration when all of the children can get together (his children are grown and out of the home) at whatever time it can be arranged, and then the kids visit grandparents and other relatives at other times. This couple has also worked cooperatively with his ex-spouses around the children's weddings and graduations, even though the feelings are not good between them. In the Nolan family, they decorate two trees every year so that both his and her children could continue in familiar patterns.

In the Hall family, Christmas is a very big event which Mrs. Hall is not willing to share with her ex-husband, Hank's father. The Halls get together with his and her extended families for a big event at Christmas. Hank's father has not complained about this arrangement. He lives out of state, so when Hank does visit, it involves travel and time. Other families who have ex-spouses out of state, however, do alternate having the children home at Christmas or Thanksgiving. In all of the families who have children away for Christmas, they celebrate the holiday together at another time. In the Wilson family, for example, both her son and his son alternate spending Christmas and Thanksgiving at their other parents' homes. So, the children both have two big dinners. The Wilsons always have a big family feast with friends and relatives at a time when his and her sons can be home. Decorating the tree and attending church are important parts of their holiday rituals. She brought into the marriage the tradition of tree decorating, and they developed together the tradition of having a big feast with music for their friends.

Two of these families have brought both Christian and Jewish traditions into the marriage. Although one family does not consider itself religious and the other family does, both families have consciously brought in traditions from both cultures. In the Allen family, her sons were baptized Catholic, while their little girl has had both Christian baptism and Jewish naming ceremonies. They celebrate holidays from both traditions as a family. They consider themselves to be a family with few rituals, but they have developed one ritual that they enjoy: every New Year the family writes down the events of the previous year, and these writings are saved as records. The Martin family also celebrates Christmas and Chanukah. She brought in the tradition of decorating a Christmas tree and they each give each other a tree ornament as a gift each year. They do not have other religious traditions. A holiday tradition they have begun as their own is to have a large New Year's open house every year.

EVERYDAY RITUALS

The regular day-in-and-day-out or week-in-and-week-out rituals were very important to most of these families, too. As with the special occasion rituals, most of the families tended to keep some from before and develop some new patterns of their own. These activities tended to be grouped around church events, sporting or music events, special meals, or special bedtime rituals, such as reading, prayers, or special hugs.

The Evans family is a good example of a family with many day-to-day rituals. This couple met through church, they were referred to this study through their church, and religion is an important theme in their family life. It is not surprising, therefore, that attending church together and activities with friends from church are important traditions for them. Mrs. Evans came from a female-headed small family with one sister. Her husband comes from a large family with several brothers, and he was used to a more rough-and-tumble family life. They are both professional people, but it was she who owned a house. He had lived with his parents since moving back to the Midwest with his son. They joke that he provided the family and she provided the house.

They each came into the family with very different life experiences and different life styles. These differences could have caused problems, but instead they have felt enriched by the other's interests and habits. He had been married twice before, and felt that she had taught him how to be a good husband, but he had been an excellent parent, and she, who had never been around children much, was a willing learner in that respect. He interested her in sports and she interested him in music. Luckily, they both shared a common philosophy of life, guided by their mutual interest in church and in professional life.

Mrs. Evans brought into the marriage the Christmas-tree-decorating tradition from her family, they both brought into the family the tradition of attending church on Sunday, and together they developed the day-to-day habits which became rituals. As a family, they have daily devotions and there are nightly story readings at Emil's bedtime. Going to bed is not a negative experience for Emil, as a result of this highly prized story time. In fact, (rarely needed) discipline for Emil is one night of no story.

This family has also developed the tradition of working out together. They ride bikes or engage in some other physical activity every weekend; this came from Mr. Evans. Emil is now taking music lessons, and Mrs. Evans's regular supervision of that activity has become their ritual together. Since both Mr. and Mrs. Evans are very busy with their various professional activities and separate friends, they have found regular and scheduled activities to be useful for them, and to help them bond as a family. They also enjoy attending music and sports events together as a family, and have developed mutual and family friends.

Most of these stepfamilies have developed ritualized activities enjoyed by family members, including special Sunday morning breakfasts together, family meetings, playing musical instruments together, annual vacations, and children's sporting or music events. In several of these families, everyone in the family attends and cheers for one child's athletic event on a regular basis. These games are often several nights a week in the summer. Friends and relatives may attend too, and special traditions have developed around going out to eat afterward, or coming back to the house for snacks.

In two families, married children kept in touch with their parents through attendance at siblings' games. One family has been fixing up an old house for several years; they believed that working on the house was a family activity that was a ritual for them. Other special traditions included apple picking every fall and celebrating a dog's birthday. Two families read Bible passages together, and several families mentioned bedtime stories and special hugs at bedtime.

SUMMARY

Hartman and Laird (1983) have said that family rituals are "regulatory patterns which help consolidate family identity and provide structure and cohesiveness" (p.320). The 20 families interviewed for this study supported this view. All of these families, in varying degrees, have consciously organized their family lives around regular activities aimed at developing cohesion among the members. In fact, it was interesting to note that the level of family activities among these families seemed higher than in other families, especially for those with teenagers. Since they are newer than biologically based families with children, they are developmentally at a different stage.

These family activities tend to be ritualized in that members are expected to attend, they occur regularly, and roles and behaviors are prescribed. Often there is symbolic meaning attached to the event. Examples include special ceremonies around trimming a Christmas tree, special bedtime rituals with Bible readings and hugs, and attending church or school activities as a family, with a meal afterward. One family makes banners and has a ceremony when a member receives an award or honor.

Many of these families had to start their own traditions. While that term implies customs handed down from previous generations, there have not been many traditions developed for stepfamilies. These families often said that they started new traditions partly because there were not ones that fit, and also because they wanted something different for their new family. Most of them also recognized the importance of keeping some old traditions and rituals in addition to developing new ones, to mark continuity as well as change. Some of the traditions, such as attending church or sporting events together, also helped these families become recognized by and integrated into the larger community. Several of these families have regular parties for their friends, integrating the new unit into support networks, and regular nights just for family activities, marking the boundary around their new family unit. While both the service and high-functioning groups had developed rituals and traditions, the high-functioning families had developed them more strongly.

Chapter 8

Suggestions for Others

In the other chapters, the larger ideas and concepts were discussed first, along with findings of others, and the stories from the families followed that discussion. In this chapter, the families' stories are told first, with a summary relating their ideas to the general concepts at the end.

At the close of each interview, a more open ended-format was used as the question was asked, "What suggestions do you have for others who are beginning a new stepfamily?" This was the question that all the families liked best. Not only were they warmed up by now, feeling more comfortable with the student and me, as well as the video camera, but this question allowed them to say what they wanted to say, with no implied correct subject matter. This question brought responses from all family members, even the shy children. In a few situations where the children were young and did not stay for the whole interview, this question was asked just before they left, and then the interview was resumed. Family members had definite ideas that they wanted to share with others. They often spoke directly into the camera, as if the recipient of the advice would listen to them directly, even though they knew the tapes would be erased after analysis. In this last part of the interview, inhibitions were down and there was more joking with each other and with us.

THE FAMILIES' ADVICE

The Wilsons, a family receiving services, were very articulate in offering suggestions. Mrs. Wilson said, "We tried to make our family a picture-post card family, where everyone is tightly knit into one unit. That was our problem; it didn't work, and we got frustrated, and it made things worse. We read about stepfamilies where it worked that way, and I don't know how they did it, perhaps they had younger children, but for us that expectation was not a useful one." She had the idea when they married that his children would come to her for permission and advice, as her son did. She realizes now that was an unrealistic expectation, and that having that expectation strained relationships in the family. She recommends premarital counseling for all family members to work out these issues in advance, and to learn what one can and can not expect. Mr. Wilson, on the other hand, thinks it would have been better to have lived together without marriage, because a legal marriage carries "too much baggage." Both Mr. and Mrs. Wilson recommend their financial plan of separate accounts; they like not having to ask each other for permission to spend money (see Chapter 5 for discussion of their plan). They suggest to others to keep a specific time for themselves as a couple. They did not allow themselves enough time to develop their couple relationship, because of busy work schedules and their own children's activities.

The Wilsons' suggestion to spend time developing the couple relationship was an idea echoed by most of these families. Mr. and Mrs. Foster stated their belief that one reason their stepfamily situation has worked so well is because they have had every other week alone without the children to develop their own relationship with each other and with their adult friends. When the children are there in the in-between weeks, they focus more on the children and on family activities. They believe that they have had the best of both worlds. The fact that this plan has been in effect since the beginning, when the children were young, has helped it to work well, because there were no other expectations. The children like the arrangement, too, because they love both parents and both stepparents, and would get lonesome, they said, if they were away from either family much longer than a week.

The Jones, like the Fosters, have every other week alone to develop couple time and to devote to their own friends and professional activities. They also like this arrangement, and believe that it helps them to give his daughter, Jessie, special time and time for more family activities in the other weeks. The Joneses and the Fosters recognize that the every-other-week plan is not feasible for many families, but they do recommend that couple time be planned in some way. Mr. Wilson's son also alternates every other week, but the Wilsons do not have time alone, because her son is home, and because there are other children out of the home. They believe that they have not scheduled enough couple time, and are now working on doing that more. The Evans do carefully schedule couple time, and they stressed its importance.

While there is not evidence that having a solid marriage ensures stepfamily satisfaction (for example, there still may be problems between children and stepparents, between stepsiblings, or the children may not be happy with the situation), most of these couples believe that it is an important variable if the family is to work at all. Mrs. Nolan stated that their solid marriage was the only thing that kept them going for the first two years, when the children were so unhappy. The general consensus among these families was that things are going to be rough at first, but a strong couple relationship gives them the strength to negotiate the other problems and to form the basis for the rest of the family to come together. Indeed, the words "patience" and "time" were used frequently by the well-functioning families as key words for new families to heed.

What did the children in these families have to say about all this? The Nolan children had several ideas. One said he would remind the children to "be respectful," and he would suggest that the stepparents develop friendships with the children, but not try to be their parents. Another said, "I would tell a friend who was about to find himself in a stepfamily that it will all work out once you get used to it–it takes time." Mr. and Mrs. Nolan noted that each of the five children had to adjust at his or her own pace, and that each adjusted differently.

Comments from other children included, "Stepparents should spend time with the kids, but don't force activities on them" (Art Allen). "Allow the kid to have special time for hugs and chats with the biological parent alone" (Maggie Martin). Maggie also said, "Don't push the step relationship–it takes time; find common ground and build on it." Jessie Jones said "Talk is best; talk it out." Other children stressed the importance of family meetings, not holding grudges, and family activities. Debbie Davis talked about the importance of flexibility, noting that her mom and stepdad moved the Christmas celebration to the twenty-third so she could have Christmas eve celebration with her father's side of the family and be with her maternal grandparents on Christmas day.

Flexibility was an idea expressed by many members of these families. Mrs. Butterworth said her first three suggestions were "flexibility, flexibility, and flexibility." She also said it is important to have a "can do" attitude, and that communication, respect, and privacy are important too. Finally, she added, "You have to learn to put up with things that you aren't used to and don't like. Talk things out, and discuss rules and expectations. Before you jump into a situation, discuss how you would have handled the situation differently."

The Allen family spent quite a bit of time offering suggestions. Mrs. Allen said that it is all right to be angry, but "talk it out and listen to each other." The family members agreed that communication and respect for each other are most important. Mrs. Allen added that the stepparent should not be too dominant at first, that it is all right to voice opinions but not to try to reshape things. They also suggested that it is sometimes helpful to move away from extended family if they are not supportive. Mr. Allen's parents did not approve of her or her children, and their relationship is easier now that they have moved across the country. However, their social network is small in their new location, and that is a stressor.

Mr. Lange said that it is important to remember that "there is no such thing as a perfect family, otherwise you frustrate yourself trying for something that is not possible." He also said that he wished he had been more patient with his children, and more giving, and he is trying that with her boys. He stressed the importance of discussing issues with the other set of parents.

Mr. Martin said, "When you're coming in as an outsider you have to learn to wait; the good parts come in spurts. Learn to rely on the strength of the couple relationship, and trust your spouse to raise his or her own children. I made the conscious decision to stay out of the mother-daughter relationship, and while it was not always easy, it was for the best and I would recommend that to others. With the stepchild, learn to respect each other by finding a common interest.

Respect and liking each other are more important than love." Mr. Martin also discussed the importance of drawing boundaries around the new unit. At first, they had a friend's child also in the home, and "things were just too fuzzy." Finding neutral territory can be important. When he moved into her house, it seemed like her house. Then, they moved to another city for his job, and it was his house. Now, they have moved again, and it feels best because it is clearly their house: parts of it look like him and parts of it look like her, and other parts are mixed or different altogether. Another suggestion from Mr. Martin's stepdaughter, Maggie, was "keep an open mind and think about something before you say it." Mr. Martin added, "Don't sweat the small stuff, don't always go with the rules, there can be another way."

Suggestions from other families included, "ability to disagree," "give all the love you can to the kids," "wait," "don't change their patterns too quickly," "have respect for each other and make time for the couple relationship," "let kids adjust at their own pace," "you have to be willing to bend," "communication, consistency, honesty, and love," and "the stepparent should make a slow transition into discipline." Last, comments about the importance of a sense of humor, not holding grudges, and being flexible were very common across most of these families.

SUMMARY

Common themes as to what works can be isolated from the suggestions. In this project, 20 stepfamilies, 83 persons, were interviewed regarding their ideas on the subject. These interviews were in-depth, in-home interviews, with all persons living in the home present. Most of these families (14 of 20) were referred by self or others as high functioning, while the other six were recruited through counseling agencies. While there were significant differences between the groups in overall functioning as measured by the Beavers and Hampson's scales (1990), the entire group of 20 families represent families that function well, in varying degrees (Kelley, 1992). See Figure 1 for distribution of family scores on the family health continuum, and Chapters 1 and 2 for discussion of those scales.

There were differences between these groups as to length of current marriage, suggesting that developing healthy stepfamilies is a process, and that time is required for integration. Furthermore, information from these families suggests that total integration should probably not be expected nor considered the desired state for stepfamilies. The importance of recognizing the developmental stages discussed in the literature (Goetting, 1982; Mills, 1984; Whiteside, 1982) were supported in this study. Because stepfamilies have children from the beginning, and because at least one parent has been married or in a couple relationship previously, there are often expectations that the new family can pick up where the previous family left off, and that is not the case. The new stepfamily is at the same developmental stage of a new couple beginning marriage, with more energy needed to go into the couple relationship and into drawing boundaries around the family as a unit. These families, even those with teenagers, spent a great deal of time in family activities, looking more like newer families with younger children, as they developed family identity. Whiteside (1982) has noted that there have been few studies of stepfamily development because most studies have been with stepfamilies who have been together less than three years. In this preliminary study, there was a wide range as to how long they had been together, and the findings regarding these factors are interesting. Many of the high-functioning families interviewed said that the first two years were the most difficult, and that time and patience were crucial.

The idea that stepfamilies are different, and need a different set of rules and expectations, was supported by this study. Most of the high-functioning families said that the old rules do not work for stepfamilies and that stepfamilies should not try to model themselves after other families. Yet, some of the principles drawn from these high-functioning stepfamilies could also apply to healthy family functioning in general.

In extracting key themes from these high-functioning families as to what works, several concepts did seem striking. First is the value of children maintaining contact with persons important to them after the parental divorce. While Furstenberg and Nord (1985) report that 75 percent of noncustodial stepfathers lose contact with their children within three years of divorce, in these families 70 percent of the children maintained contact with both biological parents, and a higher percentage than that continued to see grandparents from both sides. Cooperation with ex-spouses, with emphasis on children's welfare, was another recurring theme.

The importance of clear communication, with some planned mechanism for implementing it, was another common thread. Regular family meetings with rules discussed and agreed upon by as many people as possible were suggested and carried out in these high-functioning families, especially in the beginning stages of marriage.

Another key theme found in these families was the idea of going slowly, and allowing the family to develop at its own pace. In most of these families the stepparent did not come in as a substitute parent, but took on a different role, as spouse of the parent and gradually as friend and special person to the child. Furthermore, stepsiblings were not expected to feel like siblings at first, and love and sharing were not pushed. When stepparents came into a family of young children, they often took on parental roles of discipline and nurturing after a while, but when the children were older that plan did not work. Even in those families where the stepparents never took on disciplinary functions, a strong sense of family developed around the new units.

Another, related, theme that emerged from these interviews was the importance of respect over love in steprelationships. The expectation of instant and equal love was not present in these families, and the exceptions to that rule were in the families receiving services. In most of these families it was all right to call the stepparent by the first name, and to feel closer to and spend more time with the biological parent. One question that was not asked of these families was who took who's name. In reviewing the interview forms, however, it appears that most children kept their own surnames, except when the children were young and the biological parent was out of the picture. (In the genograms for this book, however, the family members were all given the same surnames to make it easier for the reader.) One parent reported that the child having a different name from the parents was a problem in school, so they had to change it to accommodate the school forms. In these families, the term stepmother or stepfather was not toxic; most used the term in a loving way.

The importance of the couple relationship was stressed by all of the families, but, as noted in the literature (Clingempeel, Brand, and Ievoli, 1984; White and Booth, 1985), that is not enough to ensure general stepfamily satisfaction. Whereas a strong marriage is central in establishing the foundation of the stepfamily, it is probably best not to flaunt it in front of the children. Children often assume a primary relationship with the custodial parent after a divorce, and it is natural for jealousy to occur when a stepparent comes into the picture. Several of these children expressed some jealousy, or said that there was some at first. One girl said she hated it when her dad and stepmother were "lovey dovey." The achievement of this delicate balance between giving a clear message to the children that the marriage is solid and that the adults stand behind and support each other, and yet allowing for continuing special relationships with biological children was discussed in Chapter 6, especially in regard to the Evans family. The idea of showing love but reducing physical affection in front of the children is probably a good one, especially since there may be sexual tensions in stepfamilies.

Allowing for privacy and space was a matter attended to by these families. More privacy and space are needed than in biologically based families, and many families found it useful to develop their own sense of space by moving to neutral territory.

No clear consensus emerged as to what works best for handling money, but it was clear that money management is more complicated in stepfamilies where there are different sources of money coming in and going out, and many decisions are out of the control of at least one spouse. While most of these families pooled most of their money, because it is less complicated, the families that did keep money separate found it very important that they do so.

Flexibility was probably the word heard most often when these families discussed what was important. First, there needs to be flexibility of rules. One stepfather said, "Don't stick to the rules too much, find another way." A stepmother said, "There will be things that you won't like, and you just have to get used to them." Another stepmother said, "When it comes to customs and traditions you just have to forget how things should be; things will be different." A child said, "You have to get used to different rules at different houses. For example, it is OK to eat on the sofa at one house, but it's not OK at the other house. It works out fine, you just have to remember where you are."

Stepfamilies also need to be more flexible in roles. In these families, both adults produced incomes, nurtured, disciplined, and worked around the house. Roles were divided more along the lines of who is the biological parent than who is male or female. The children also tended to be more flexible in household chores. The rule here seemed to be "Do whatever needs to be done or whatever is asked." There was also flexibility as to who went to whom about what, and there was more boundary flexibility; children were often moving back and forth between two homes, yet felt a part of both families.

Last, a common theme found in these families, and especially in the high-functioning families, was the ability to have fun together, not taking things too seriously and having a sense of humor. The interviews generally were fun with good humor prevailing, and many families even laughed over the problematic situations that they had encountered. In only three families was the atmosphere serious and problem focused, and they were all families receiving services.

Many families discussed how the expectations to be like a first-married family had caused problems in the beginning, and recommended more information for stepfamilies. At the end of this book, there is a list of readings about stepfamilies that may be useful for families and for persons working with stepfamilies. Many of those books have come out since this project was begun, suggesting that the topic is beginning to be addressed more fully.

Suggestions and themes from these families that would be useful for families in general include flexibility, clear communication, decreased sex role stereotyping, fun and good humor, and strong social and community support systems. In stepfamilies, however, these ideas assume extra importance. Themes from these families suggesting differences included discipline and nurturing from one, not both, of the adults in the home, more cross-generational alliances, more permeable boundaries allowing for children to move back and forth between homes without feeling out of the system, inequality of parental roles, and somewhat different resources and rules for different sets within the family.

Finally, stories from these families demonstrate that stepfamilies are different, but they are not necessarily problematic. In fact, all of these families are very high functioning. Even though stepfamilies may function at very high levels, they generally need to allow for adjustment time, especially for complex stepfamilies. Further, they need to develop rules and structures that fit them, which may be different from the expectations of biological families.

References

Ahrons, C. R. 1979. The binuclear family: Two households, one family. *Alternative Lifestyles* 2:499-515.

Ahrons, C. R. 1981. The continuing coparental relationship between divorced spouses. *American Journal of Orthopsychiatry* 51:315-328.

Ahrons, C. R., and R. H. Rodgers. 1987. *Divorced families*. New York: W. W. Norton.

Ahrons, C. R., and L. Wallisch. 1987. Parenting in the binuclear family: Relationships between biological and step parents. In *Remarriage and stepfamilies: Research and theory*, edited by K. Pasley and M. Ihinger-Tallman. New York: Guilford Press.

Beavers, W. R., and R. B. Hampson. 1990. *Successful families: Assessment and intervention*. New York: W. W. Norton.

Bernstein, A. C. 1989. *Yours, mine, and ours: How families change when remarried parents have a child together*. New York: Charles Scribner's Sons.

Bohannan, P., and H. Yahraes. 1979. Stepfathers as parents. In *Families today: A research sampler on families and children*, edited by E. Corfman. Washington, D.C.: U.S. Government Printing Office.

Brown, A. C. 1986. Factors associated with family functioning in non-counseling and counseling stepfamilies. Unpublished dissertation. California Graduate School of Marital and Family Therapy, San Rafael, California.

Carter, B. 1989. Clinical work with step-families. In *Building bridges: Creating balance*. 47th Annual Conference of the American Association for Marriage and Family Therapy, San Francisco.

Clingempeel, W. G., and E. Brand. 1985. Quasi-kin relationships, structural complexity, and marital quality in stepfamilies: A replication, extension, and clinical implications. *Family Relations* 34:401-409.

Clingempeel, W. G., E. Brand, and R. Ievoli. 1984. Stepparent-stepchild relationships in stepmother and stepfather families: A multimethod study. *Family Relations* 33:465-473.

Clingempeel, W. G., and S. Segal. 1986. Stepparent-stepchild relationships and the psychological adjustment of children in stepmother and stepfather families. *Child Development* 57(2):474-484.

Coleman, M., L. H. Ganong, and R. Gingrich. 1985. Stepfamily strengths: A review of popular literature. *Family Relations 34*: 583-589.

Crohn, H., C. J. Sager, H. Brown, E. Rodstein, and L. Walker. 1982. A basis for understanding and treating the remarried family. In *Therapy with remarriage families*, edited by J. C. Hansen and L. Messinger. Rockville, MD: Aspen Publications.

Dahl, A. S., K. M. Cowgill, and R. Asmundsson. 1987. Life in remarriage families. *Social Work, 32*(1):40-44.

Duberman, L. 1975. *The reconstituted family: A study of remarried couples and their children.* Chicago: Nelson Hall.

Epstein, N. B., L. M. Baldwin, and D. S. Bishop. 1983. The McMaster family assessment device. *Journal of Marital and Family Therapy 9*(2):171-180.

Epstein, N. B., D. S. Bishop, and L. M. Baldwin. 1982. McMaster model of family functioning: A view of the normal family. In *Normal family processes*, edited by F. Walsh. New York: Guilford Press.

Epstein, N. B., D. S. Bishop, and S. Levin. 1978. The McMaster model of family functioning. *Journal of Marriage and Family Counseling 4*:19-31.

Fiese, B. H. 1992. Dimensions of family rituals across two generations: Relation to adolescent identity. *Family Process 31*(2): 151-162.

Furstenberg, F. F., and C. W. Nord. 1985. Parenting apart: Patterns of childrearing after marital disruption. *Journal of Marriage and the Family 47*(4):893-904.

Ganong, L. H., and M. Coleman. 1986. A comparison of clinical and empirical literature on children in stepfamilies. *Journal of Marriage and the Family 48*:309-318.

Giles-Sims, J. 1984. The stepparent role. *Journal of Family Issues 15*:116-130.

Glick, P. C., and Sung-Lin Lin. 1986. Recent changes in divorce and remarriage. *Journal of Marriage and Family Therapy 48*:737-747.

Goetting, A. 1982. The six stations of remarriage: Developmental tasks of remarriage after divorce. *Family Relations 31*:213-222.

Guerin, P., L. Fay, S. Burden, and J. Kautto. 1987. *The evaluation and treatment of marital conflict: A four stage approach.* New York: Basic Books.

Hartin, W. W. 1990. Re-marriage: Some issues for clients and therapists. *A. N. Z. Journal of Family Therapy 11*:36-42.

Hartman, A., and J. Laird. 1983. *Family-centered social work practice.* New York: Free Press.

Hetherington, E. 1979. Divorce: A child's perspective. *American Psychologist 34*:851-858.

Hetherington, E. M., M. Cox, and R. Cox. 1985. Long-term effects of divorce and remarriage on the adjustment of children. *Journal of the American Academy of Child Psychiatry 24*(5):518-530.

Hetherington, E. M., M. Stanley-Hagen, and E. R. Anderson. 1989. Marital transitions: A child's perspective. *American Psychologist 44*(2):303-312.

Ihinger-Tallman, M., and K. Pasley. 1986. Remarriage and integration within the community. *Journal of Marriage and the Family 48*:395-405.

Imber-Black, E. 1988. *Families and larger systems: A family therapist's guide through the labyrinth.* New York: Gilford Press.

Johnson, H. C. 1980. Working with stepfamilies: Principles of practice. *Social Work 25*:304-308.

Kelley, P. 1992. Healthy stepfamily functioning. *Families in Society 73*(10):579-587.

Kelley, P., V. Kelley, and B. Williams. 1989. Treatment of adolescents: A comparison of individual and family therapy. *Social Casework 70*(8):461-468.

Knaub, P. K., S. L. Hanna, and N. Stinnett. 1984. Strengths of remarried families. *Journal of Divorce 7*(3):41-55.

Kurdek, L. A. 1989. Relationship quality for newly married husbands and wives: Marital history, stepchildren, and individual-difference predictors. *Journal of Marriage and the Family 51*:1053-1064.

Letters: Child-support face-off. 1992. *Newsweek* (May):12-14.

McCubbin, H. J., J. Patterson, J. C. Comeau, J. Constance, and E. A. Kauble. 1981. Family stress, coping, and social support: Recent research and theory. In *Systematic assessment of family stress, resources, and coping*, edited by K. Davidson. St. Paul, MN: Family Stress and Coping Project.

McGoldrick, M., and B. Carter. 1988. Forming a remarried family. In *The changing family life cycle: A framework for family therapy*, 2nd ed., edited by B. Carter, and M. McGoldrick. New York: Gardner Press.

Maglin, N., and N. Schniedewind, eds. 1989. *Women and stepfamilies: Voices of anger and love*. Philadelphia: Temple University Press.

Messinger, L. 1976. Remarriage between divorced people with children from previous marriages: A proposal for preparation for marriage. *Journal of Marriage and Family Counseling* 2:193-200.

Mills, D. M. 1984. A model for stepfamily development. *Family Relations 33*:365-372.

Minuchin, S. 1974. *Families and family therapy*. Cambridge, MA: Harvard University Press.

Nunn, G. D., T. S. Parish, and R. J. Worthing. 1983. Perceptions of personal and familial adjustment by children from intact, single-parent, and reconstituted families. *Psychology in the Schools 20*(2):166-174.

Olson, D. H., D. H. Sprenkle, and C. S. Russell. 1979. Circumplex model of marital and family systems: 1. Cohesion and adaptability dimensions, family types, and clinical applications. *Family Process 18*(1):3-26.

Orleans, M., B. J. Palisi, and D. Caddell. 1989. Marriage adjustment and satisfaction of stepfathers: Their feelings and perceptions of decision making and stepchildren relations. *Family Relations 38*:371-377.

Oxford American Dictionary. 1980. New York: Avon Books.

Peterson, J. L., and N. Zill. 1986. Marital disruption, parent-child relationships, and behavior problems in children. *Journal of Marriage and the Family 48*:245-307.

Poppen, W. A., and P. N. White. 1984. Transition to the blended family. *Elementary School Guidance and Counseling 19*:50-61.

Roberts, J. 1988. Setting the frame: Definition, functions, and typology of rituals. In *Rituals in families and family therapy*, edited by E. Imber-Black, J. Roberts, and R. A. Whiting. New York: W. W. Norton.

Robinson, B. E. 1984. The contemporary American stepfather. *Family Relations 33*:381-388.

Robinson, M. 1980. Step-families: A reconstituted family system. *Journal of Family Therapy 2*:45-69.

Sager, J. W., H. S. Brown, H. Crohn, T. Engel, E. Rodstein, and L. Walker. 1983. *Treating the remarried family.* New York: Brunner/Mazel.

Santrock, J. W., R. Warshak, C. Lindbergh, and L. Meadows. 1982. Children's and parents' observed social behavior in stepfather families. *Child Development 53*:472-480.

Schwebel, A., M. Fine, and M. Renner. 1991. A study of perceptions of the step parent role. *Journal of Family Issues 12*:43-57.

Stern, P. N. 1978. Stepfather families: Integration around child discipline. *Issues in Mental Health Nursing 1*(2):49-56.

Visher, E. B., and J. S. Visher. 1979. *Stepfamilies: A guide to working with stepparents and stepchildren.* New York: Brunner/Mazel.

Visher, E. B., and J. S. Visher. 1982. *How to win as a stepfamily.* New York: Dembner Books.

Visher, E. B., and J. S. Visher. 1985. Stepfamilies are different. *Journal of Family Therapy 7*(1):9-18.

Visher, E. B., and J. S. Visher. 1988. *Old loyalties, new ties: Therapeutic strategies with stepfamilies.* New York: Brunner/Mazel.

Wallerstein, J. S. 1985. Children of divorce: Preliminary report of a ten year follow-up of older children and adolescents. *Journal of the American Academy of Child Psychiatry 24*:545-553.

Wallerstein, J. S. and J. B. Kelly. 1980. *Surviving the break up: How children and parents cope with divorce.* New York: Basic Books.

Webster's new twentieth century dictionary of the English language. 1980. New York: William Collins Publishers.

White, L. K., and A. Booth. 1985. The quality and stability of remarriages: The role of step children. *American Sociological Review 50*:689-698.

Whiteside, M. F. 1982. Remarriage: A family developmental process. *Journal of Marital and Family Therapy 8*(2):59-68.

Whitsett, D., and H. Land. 1992. Role strain, coping, and marital satisfaction of stepparents. *Families in Society 73*(2):79-92.

Other Books on the Subject

The following references are offered as an aid to families, educators, therapists, and others wanting to understand more about stepfamilies. These are but a few of the many good books on the subject. Since many of the books listed below have extensive bibliographies, they can be consulted for information about further reading. This list was developed by Lary Belman, MSW Candidate, University of Iowa, and Beth Larsen, MSW Clinical Social Worker, Delacrest Mental Health Center, Manchester, IA.

Beer, W. R. 1992. *American stepfamilies*. New Brunswick, NJ: Transaction Publishers.

Beer, W. R. 1989. *Strangers in the house: The World of stepsiblings and halfsiblings*. New Brunswick, NJ: Transaction Books.

Berman, C. 1986. *Making it as a stepparent: New roles/new rules*. New York: Harper & Row.
A "how-to" book that looks at how to prevent or resolve problems. It takes an encouraging look at the potential rewards of stepfamily life.

Bernstein, A. C. 1989. *Yours, mine, and ours: How families change when remarried parents have a child together*. New York: Scribner.
The author summarizes the findings of a study representing 55 remarried households regarding the effects of a mutual child in a stepfamily.

Burns, C. 1985. *Stepmotherhood: How to survive without feeling frustrated, left out, or wicked*. New York: Times Books.
Deals with the unique problems of stepmothers. It is based on extensive interviews with more than 40 stepmothers who have spoken frankly about their experiences in this difficult role. Their

stories, along with the author's analysis and understanding of them, can be helpful to women who are about to become stepmothers and to those who already are. The book suggests solutions to many stepmothering problems and advice on how to live with what is beyond the stepmother's control.

Burt, M., ed. 1989. *Stepfamilies stepping ahead.* Lincoln, NE: The Stepfamily Association of America.
A workbook for stepfamilies themselves to use; a good book for counselors and clergy to give or loan to newly forming step parents. Particularly valuable is a concluding section by Emily Visher describing eight behavioral steps adults can take to help to integrate the new stepfamily. The cost is $9.95 plus shipping.

Coleman, M., and L. H. Ganong. 1988. *Bibliotherapy with stepchildren.* Springfield, IL: C. C. Thomas.
Useful for stepfamilies or anyone working with them. After a brief discussion of stepfamily concerns, the authors show how fiction and self-help books can be used to help children and adolescents in stepfamilies. Included is a review of 265 fiction and self-help books.

Dinkmeyer, D., G. D. McKay, and J. L. McKay. 1992. *New beginnings: Skills for single parents and stepfamily parents.* Champaign, IL: Research Press.
Focuses on the needs of stepfamilies and single parents. Parent trainers and family therapists, as well as their clients, will find this a practical parenting manual. Some of the useful areas that this book explores are bonds of preexisting relationships, managing conflicts between spouses on different disciplining styles, and directing family meetings.

Evans, M. D. 1986. *This is me and my two families.* New York: Magination Press.
A workbook for children and adults to improve understanding through talking, writing, and art. Exercises encourage communication and expression of feelings that improve understanding about divorce and remarriage.

Hughes, C. 1991. *Stepparents: Wicked or wonderful?: An indepth study of stepparenthood.* Brookfield, VT: Gower.

Ihinger-Tallman, M. 1987. *Remarriage.* Newbury Park: Sage Publications.

Keshet, J. K. 1987. *Love and power in the stepfamily.* New York: McGraw-Hill.

Maglin, N. B., and N. Schniedewind. eds. 1989. *Women and stepfamilies: Voices of anger and love.* Philadelphia: Temple University Press.

A book about stepmothers based on interviews with more than 30 women and on research about the cultural meaning of stepmothering. It deals with who stepmothers are, how they have been portrayed in literature and folk tales, what society expects of them, and what they expect of themselves. The history of stepmothering is traced through the work of a selection of writers, and, to illuminate some of the problems of the stepmother, a few clinical studies are included about stepmothers who suffer stress and depression in relation to their stepmothering roles.

Martin, D., and, M. Martin. 1992. *Stepfamilies in therapy.* San Francisco, CA: Jossey-Bass.

Designed to help the human services professional understand stepfamilies and help them build a healthy and stable family life. It examines the complex issues facing stepfamilies, such as grief over divorce, negative stereotypes of stepfamilies, child custody and visitation disputes, unrealistic expectations of family life, and confusing relationships with the extended family. Therapeutic approaches, strategies, and interventions for effective assessment and treatment are offered.

Relative strangers: Studies of stepfamily processes. 1988. Totowa, NJ: Rowman and Littlefield.

Smith, D. 1990. *Stepmothering.* New York: Harvester/Wheatsheaf.

Interviews with thirty stepmothers. The book discusses stepmothering from personal points of view to their representation in literature, including expectations of society and self.

Stepfamily Association of America, 215 Centential Mall South, Suite 212, Lincoln, NE 68508 (800-735-0329).

An organization which provides helpful information for people considering becoming step parents and for those who are already step parents. It provides information and advocacy for stepfamilies: self-help programs through local chapters, educational resources, a quarterly bulletin, an annual national conference, and chapter start-up information. This information is a valuable resource for obtaining information about stepfamilies.

Visher, E., and J. S. Visher. 1980. *Stepfamilies: Myths and realities.* Secaucus, NJ: Citadel Press.

Visher, E., and J. S. Visher. 1982. *How to win as a stepfamily.* New York: Dembner Books.
Contains information and suggestions for adults on how to make their stepfamilies work. There are numerous personal anecdotes illustrating a variety of challenges and their successful mastery. Among the topics the book addresses are such troublesome issues as dealing with former spouses and new grandparents, legal issues involving custody, visitation, adoption, and money, feelings of loss, and the need for flexibility. The book demonstrates that stepfamilies can be good families in which to raise children and find personal satisfaction and growth.

Visher, E., and J. S. Visher. 1988. *Old loyalties, new ties: Therapeutic strategies with stepfamilies.* New York: Brunner/Mazel.
A problem-oriented book that covers basic theoretical concepts that will be helpful to stepfamily adults as well as to therapists and counselors. It deals with therapeutic strategies that will be useful to professional helpers in dealing with, for example, loyalty conflicts, boundary problems, power issues, and closeness and distance. In a closing section, the authors discuss the ways in which they view stepfamily therapy as differing from therapeutic work with nuclear families.

Index